GABA AND GLUTAMATE - NEW DEVELOPMENTS IN NEUROTRANSMISSION RESEARCH

Edited by **Janko Samardzic**

GABA And Glutamate - New Developments In Neurotransmission Research
http://dx.doi.org/10.5772/intechopen.68762
Edited by Janko Samardzic

Contributors

Arturo Ortega, Esther Lopez-Bayghen, Carla Angulo-Rojo, Dinorah Hernandez-Melchor, Bruno Lopez-Bayghen, Leticia Ramirez, Gabriela Beatriz Acosta, Christiane Hampe, Mario Manto, Hiroshi Mitoma, Sunitha P Kumaran, Janko Samardzic, Ing-Feng Chang, Shashi Singh, Graham Johnston, Tina Hinton

Published by InTech
Janeza Trdine 9, 51000 Rijeka, Croatia

Publishing Process Manager Marina Dusevic
Technical Editor SPi Global
Cover InTech Design team

First published March, 2018
Printed in Croatia
Legal deposit, Croatia: National and University Library in Zagreb

Additional hard copies can be obtained from orders@intechopen.com

GABA And Glutamate - New Developments In Neurotransmission Research, Edited by Janko Samardzic
p. cm.
Print ISBN 978-953-51-3821-1
Online ISBN 978-953-51-3822-8

For EU product safety concerns:
IN TECH d.o.o., Prolaz Marije Krucifikse Kozulić 3, 51000 Rijeka, Croatia, info@intechopen.com or visit our website at intechopen.com.

Meet the editor

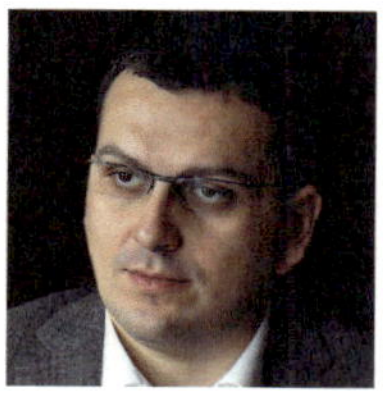

Dr. Janko Samardzic is an Assistant Professor and Clinical Pharmacologist at the Medical Faculty of the University of Belgrade in Serbia. He holds a PhD in Medical Pharmacology and has an extensive experience and expertise in Basic and Applied Neuroscience. Dr. Samardzic completed his postdoctoral studies at the University KU Leuven, Belgium and postgraduate courses at the Erasmus University Medical Center in Rotterdam, the Netherlands. He also holds the position of Visiting Fellow at the University Children's Hospital Basel, Switzerland. Dr. Samardzic is a member of the European College of Neuropsychopharmacology, Austrian Pharmacological Society, Swiss Society of Clinical Pharmacology and Toxicology, and Serbian Pharmacological Society. He is the author of many peer-reviewed papers and a frequent speaker at international scientific conferences.

Contents

Preface

The inhibition and excitation of neural networks form the basis of information transfer in the mammalian central nervous system. The key to most complex brain processes lies in the adequate balance between inhibitory and excitatory actions of amino acid neurotransmitters. The dominant inhibitory neurotransmitter is gamma-aminobutyric acid (GABA), while the principal excitatory neurotransmitter is glutamate. Furthermore, an increase or a decrease in their activity is associated with a number of neurological and psychiatric diseases. The following seven chapters provide the reader with an overview of the latest research/review data on GABA/glutamate system organization and function, receptor structure, subtypes and their ligands, as well as translational approaches and clinical implications.

The introductory chapter describes the basic functioning and the relevance of GABA/glutamate balance in the normal brain functioning, focusing on the role of their receptors. The second chapter, titled "Early Life Experience: Maternal Separation, Involvement of GABA and Glutamate Transporters," summarizes scientific data and opinion regarding maternal separation as a model of early life experience of postnatal stress, with focus on the involvement of GABA and glutamate transporters. The third chapter, "Notch Signaling in the Astroglial Phenotype: Relevance to Glutamatergic Transmission," addresses issues related to the role of notch signaling in radial glia, with emphasis on glial glutamate transporter regulation as a key element in the molecular mechanisms that support glutamatergic neurotransmission. "Pharmacological Studies with Specific Agonist and Antagonist of Animal iGluR on Root Growth in *Arabidopsis thaliana*" presents original data from a pharmacology-based functional study of ionotropic glutamate receptors (iGluRs) in plants, suggesting a correlation between the putative iGluR-like channel function and the modification of root growth and development in the Arabidopsis roots. This is followed by a very up-to-date review titled "GABA and Glutamate: Their Transmitter Role in the CNS and Pancreatic Islets," in which the authors address not only the role of both neurotransmitters during development but also the extra-neuronal glutamatergic and GABAergic signaling in pancreatic islets of Langerhans, and possible associations with type 1 diabetes mellitus. Further clinical implications are discussed in the sixth chapter titled "Antagonists of Ionotropic Receptors for the Inhibitory Neurotransmitter GABA: Therapeutic Indications." The authors examine the antagonism of ionotropic GABA receptors, reflecting on the use of GABA receptor antagonists in the last 10 years and their possible therapeutic potential. Finally, the chapter "Clinical Applications of MR Spectroscopy (MRS) in Neurosciences" delivers a detailed description of the methodology and the relevance of MRS as an important diagnostic and research tool in clinical neuroscience.

Therefore, the book offers readers a rich collection of data regarding current and future applications of GABA and glutamate neurotransmission, including promising research strategies and potential clinical benefits.

Janko Samardzic MD, PhD, Ass. Prof.
Institute of Pharmacology, Clinical Pharmacology and Toxicology
Medical Faculty, University of Belgrade, Serbia

Chapter 1

Introductory Chapter: GABA/Glutamate Balance: A Key for Normal Brain Functioning

Janko Samardzic, Dragana Jadzic, Boris Hencic,
Jasna Jancic and Dubravka Svob Strac

Additional information is available at the end of the chapter

http://dx.doi.org/10.5772/intechopen.74023

1. Introduction

The basis of information transfer in the mammalian central nervous system (CNS) consists of excitation and inhibition of neuronal networks. The messengers responsible for propagating these excitatory and inhibitory actions are amino acid neurotransmitters [1]. The principal excitatory neurotransmitter is glutamate, while the principle inhibitory neurotransmitter is gamma-aminobutyric acid (GABA). Coordination between these two principal neurotransmitters ensures adequate rhythmic activity, which may involve either a single neuron or multiple neuronal groups, thus altering synaptic plasticity and ensuring a normal functioning of CNS [2]. As this spatiotemporal framework of different patterns in neural oscillations is essential for information processing throughout the brain [3], the deviations in normal activity of either system or their interactions are associated with a number of neurological and psychiatric diseases [4].

The GABA/glutamate functional balance could be achieved by homeostatic control of presynaptic elements such as glutamate and GABA release, which could be the result of changes in their metabolism (synthesis or degradation involving various enzymes), compartmentation, and recycling (involving plasma transporters) and in the amounts of transmitters available for release from synaptic vesicles (involving vesicular transporters). However, it is generally considered that homeostatic plasticity mechanisms in the brain are mediated primarily by regulation of expression and function of glutamate and GABA receptors [5].

2. GABA and its receptors

Every third chemical synapse in the brain uses neurotransmitter GABA as an integral part of the neurotransmission process. GABA mediates its effects via two types of receptors: ionotropic $GABA_A$ and metabotropic $GABA_B$ receptors [6]. Although a third type of GABA receptor with pharmacological specificities has been identified, the term $GABA_C$ has not received broad consensus among experts. Additionally, the International Union of Basic and Clinical Pharmacology (IUPHAR) has classified $GABA_C$ as a type of $GABA_A$ receptor [7].

$GABA_A$ receptors generally contain chloride ion channels but can, in varying degrees, also contain calcium, sodium, and potassium channels. $GABA_A$ receptors mediate the majority of GABA inhibitory actions in the CNS [4]. They are pentameric transmembrane receptors made up of 5 subunit proteins that form an ion channel selectively permeable to chloride anions. Although mainly localized on postsynaptic membranes, they can also be found extrasynaptically, especially $GABA_A$ receptors containing $\alpha4$, $\alpha5$, or $\alpha6$ subunits [8]. Unexpectedly, $GABA_A$ receptors have also been found on glial cells, potentially providing adaptational support for adjacent neurons [9]. Activation of $GABA_A$ receptors leads to a change in the conformational state of associated ion channels, resulting in increased permeability to chloride ions. GABAergic mechanisms are also involved in metabolic processes [10], and a negative correlation between the intensity of GABAergic neurotransmission and metabolic processes in cerebral tissue has been established. So far, 19 subunits of $GABA_A$ receptors have been cloned and classified into several structurally related subfamilies (α 1–6, β 1–3, γ 1–3, δ, ε, θ, π, ϱ 1–3). The most frequently found $GABA_A$ receptor composition is an aggregate composed of two α, two β, and one γ subunit [4]. Receptors that, in addition to two α and two β subunits, contain some other non-γ subunit are rare. Receptors composed only of α and β isoforms also exist. The subunit composition determines the functional and pharmacological properties of $GABA_A$ receptors. For example, $\alpha1$ $GABA_A$ receptors mediate sedative and anticonvulsant actions, whereas the $\alpha2$ subunit is responsible for anxiolytic action of benzodiazepines. Zolpidem, a commonly prescribed sedative for sleep initiation, has a high binding affinity for $GABA_A$ receptors containing the $\alpha1$ subunit [11].

GABA action through $GABA_A$ receptors results in chloride channel opening and increased postsynaptic membrane permeability. In addition to the well-determined benzodiazepine binding site, at least 13 different and structurally specific sites on the $GABA_A$ receptors have been identified: (1) GABA and other agonist-binding sites, as well as competitive antagonists; (2) picrotoxin site near ion channel; (3) barbiturates binding site; (4) neuroactive steroids binding site; (5) ethanol binding site; (6) inhalation anesthetics stereoselective binding sites; (7) furosemide diuretic binding site; (8) Zn^{2+} ion binding site; (9) other divalent cation binding sites; (10) La^{3+} ions site; (11) sites for phosphorylation of specific protein kinases; (12) phospholipid-binding sites; and (13) sites involved in interaction of $GABA_A$ receptor and microtubules, which promote receptor grouping on postsynaptic membranes [12]. Modulators of $GABA_A$ receptor complex interact with these binding sites in three possible ways: positive allosteric modulators that potentiate chloride ion flux (agonists), negative modulators that reduce GABA-induced chloride ion flux (inverse agonists), and neutral allosteric modulators that competitively block the effects of these two types of agonists-antagonists.

On the other hand, $GABA_B$ metabotropic receptors, characterized by stereoselective ligand (−) baclofen, belong to the seven transmembrane G-protein-coupled receptor superfamily. They are pre- and postsynaptic G-protein-coupled receptors that negatively modulate adenylyl cyclase and inositol triphosphate synthesis. Heterodimeric structure as a result of GABAB1 and GABAB2 subunit assembly is necessary for appropriate $GABA_B$ receptor function. The extracellular domain of the GABAB1 subunit contains GABA-binding site, whereas GABAB2 subunit is important for the interaction with the G-proteins. $GABA_B$ receptor activation produces a cascade of signals that result in activation and/or inhibition of voltage-dependent calcium channels. $GABA_B$ receptor is located both centrally and peripherally, particularly in the thalamus, brain stem nuclei, and spinal cord. Depending on the localization of $GABA_B$ receptors, GABA-mediated inhibitory influences can be potentiated (postsynaptic receptors, presynaptic heteroreceptors on glutamatergic endings) or reduced (autoreceptors) [13, 14]. GABAB receptor function affects behavior, learning, and memory, and therefore their pharmacological targeting may be beneficial in various neuropsychiatric disorders [15, 16].

3. Glutamate and its receptors

Glutamate, the most abundant neurotransmitter in vertebrates and precursor of GABA, is present in over 90% of all synaptic connections in the human brain and is essential for a wide variety of functions [17]. Over 20 types of mammalian glutamate receptors exist, generally classified into two main categories: voltage-sensitive (ionotropic) and ligand-sensitive (metabotropic) receptors. Ionotropic receptor channels are formed from various protein subunits assembled in heterotetrameric or homotetrameric receptors. The three types of ionotropic receptors are N-methyl-D-aspartate (NMDA), α-amino-3-hydroxy-5-methyl-4-isoxazolepropionic acid (AMPA), and kainic acid receptors. The discovery of these agonists, after which the receptors were originally named, led to the detection of other receptor agonists and antagonists [18].

The binding of glutamate to NMDA receptors (NMDARs) results in the opening of a nonselective cation channel. The opening and closing of the channel are primarily gated by ligand binding but are also voltage-dependent. Extracellular magnesium and zinc ions can bind to specific sites on the receptor, blocking the passage of other cations through the open ion channel. However, depolarization of the neuronal cell dislodges and repels these ions from the pore, therefore allowing a voltage-dependent influx of sodium and calcium ions and efflux of potassium ions [19]. The NMDA receptor is primarily a ligand-gated channel, but it does display weaker voltage-dependent modulation of the ligand-dependent gating. NMDA requires co-activation by two ligands: glutamate and either D-serine or glycine [20]. Furthermore, NMDA receptors are divided into subtypes, depending on their intracellular protein structure, NR1, NR2, and NR3. NR1 consists of eight different subunits originating from a single gene via alternative splicing. NR2 has four subunits (A–D), and NR3 has two subunits (A and B). NMDA receptors are highly expressed on both neurons and astrocytes [21]. NMDA signaling is crucial for learning, memory, recovery from injury, and brain plasticity. It is especially important for proper functioning of the hippocampus [22]. In pathological circumstances, overactivation of NMDA receptors can lead to excitotoxicity, involved in some neurodegenerative disorders such as Alzheimer's, Parkinson's, and Huntington's disease [23–25].

AMPA receptors (AMPAR) are composed of four types of subunits, designated as GluA1, GluA2, GluA3, and GluA4 [26]. These receptors are heterotetrameric, containing GluA2 and either GluA1, GluA3, or GluA4 subunits in a "dimer of dimers" structure [27, 28]. Each AMPAR consists of four subunits which make up four binding sites to which an agonist (such as glutamate) can bind. The channel opens when two binding sites are simultaneously occupied, and the current increases as more binding sites become occupied [29]. Once opened, the channel may undergo rapid desensitization and current termination. Since AMPARs open and close quickly (1 ms), they are responsible for fast excitatory synaptic transmission in the CNS [30]. The GluA2 subunit regulates whether the AMPAR is permeable to calcium and other cations, such as sodium and potassium. If receptor does not contain a GluA2, the AMPAR will be permeable to calcium, sodium, and potassium. Both NMDA and AMPA ion channels are important for plasticity and synaptic transmission at many postsynaptic membranes.

Kainate receptors (KAR) are heteromeric receptors assembled from four subunits, formerly referred to as GluR5, GluR6, GluR7, KA1, and KA2 but now named GluK1, GluK2, GluK3, GluK4, and GluK5, and grouped into low affinity (GluK1–3) and high affinity (GluK4–5) receptors. Each subunit has a large extracellular N-terminal domain, four helical transmembrane domains (M1–M4), and an intracellular C-terminal domain. GluK1–3 subunits can form both homomeric and heteromeric receptors, but GluK4 and GluK5 subunits can form only heteromeric functional ion channels together with GluK1–3 subunits. Despite their ion channel structure, KAR can also activate metabotropic signaling through noncanonical G-protein-coupled cascade. They are widely distributed in the brain and can be localized at pre-, post-, and/or extrasynaptic sites. Although KAR are less studied than AMPAR or NMDAR, it is not known that they are multifunctional neuronal modulators which play significant roles in health and disease [31].

Metabotropic glutamate receptors (mGluR) have a G-protein-linked receptor structure consisting of seven transmembrane domains with an extracellular N-terminal and an intracellular COOH terminal. When glutamate binds to a metabotropic receptor, it activates a postsynaptic intracellular G-protein, which eventually results in the opening of a membrane channel for signal transmission. Furthermore, G protein activation also triggers functional changes in the cytoplasm, resulting in gene expression and protein synthesis. For this reason, mGluR is generally considered slower acting channels than the ionotropic glutamate receptors. To date, three groups of mGluR exist. Group I receptors are coupled with phospholipase C, producing diacylglycerol and inositol triphosphate as second messengers. They are mainly expressed on the postsynaptic membrane. Group I receptors are involved in learning and memory, addiction, motor regulation, and Fragile X syndrome [32]. Groups II and III are negatively coupled to adenylyl cyclase. Impaired functioning of group II metabotropic receptors has been linked to anxiety, schizophrenia, and Alzheimer's disease. Group III metabotropic receptors also inhibit neurotransmitter release but are positioned presynaptically. They are found within the hippocampus and hypothalamus and may play a role in Parkinson's disease and anxiety disorders [33].

4. Conclusion and clinical implications

The adequate coordination of GABA and glutamate is essential to the normal functioning for the most complex brain processes. Decreased or increased GABA activity is associated with a number of neurological and psychiatric diseases. The GABAergic synapse is the site of action of several different classes of drugs that modulate inhibitory neurotransmission and are used in the pharmacotherapy of anxiety and sleep disorders, epilepsy, alcohol withdrawal, and induction and maintenance of anesthesia [34]. Moreover, glutamate dysfunction is also correlated with a wide range of nervous system disorders, such as Alzheimer's disease, and neuropsychiatric disorders, including schizophrenia, pain disorders, drug addiction, and traumatic brain and spinal cord injuries [35]. Given the importance of equilibrium of these two systems for neuronal excitability, synaptic plasticity, and cognitive functions such as learning and memory, as well as its involvement in the mood, feeding behavior, reproductive functions, pain sensitivity, aging, etc. [36], it is not surprising that the development of current and prospective pharmaceuticals, including anxiolytics, antidepressants, antipsychotics, antiepileptics, antidementia, and many other drugs, relies increasingly on GABA/glutamate balance.

Acknowledgements

Janko Samardzic's and Jasna Jancic's work has been supported by the Ministry of Education, Science and Technological Development of the Republic of Serbia (Grant nos. 175076 and 175031). The authors declare that there are no competing interests regarding the publication of this chapter.

Author details

Janko Samardzic[1*], Dragana Jadzic[2], Boris Hencic[1], Jasna Jancic[3] and Dubravka Svob Strac[4]

*Address all correspondence to: jankomedico@yahoo.es

1 Institute of Pharmacology, Clinical Pharmacology and Toxicology, Medical Faculty, University of Belgrade, Belgrade, Serbia

2 Department of Biomedical Sciences, Neuropsychopharmacology Sect, University of Cagliari, Cagliari, Italy

3 Clinic of Neurology and Psychiatry for Children and Youth, Medical Faculty, University of Belgrade, Belgrade, Serbia

4 Laboratory for Molecular Neuropsychiatry, Division of Molecular Medicine, Rudjer Boskovic Institute, Zagreb, Croatia

References

[1] Petroff OA. GABA and glutamate in the human brain. The Neuroscientist. 2002;**8**(6):562-573

[2] Foster AC, Kemp JA. Glutamate- and GABA-based CNS therapeutics. Current Opinion in Pharmacology. 2006;**6**(1):7-17

[3] Buzsaki G, Draguhn A. Neuronal oscillations in cortical networks. Science. 2004; **304**(5679):1926-1929

[4] Jacob TC, Moss SJ, Jurd R. GABA(A) receptor trafficking and its role in the dynamic modulation of neuronal inhibition. Nature Reviews. Neuroscience. 2008;**9**(5):331-343

[5] Erickson JD, De Gois S, Varoqui H, Schafer MK, Weihe E. Activity-dependent regulation of vesicular glutamate and GABA transporters: A means to scale quantal size. Neurochemistry International. 2006;**48**(6-7):643-649

[6] Chebib M, Johnston GA. The 'ABC' of GABA receptors: A brief review. Clinical and Experimental Pharmacology & Physiology. 1999;**26**(11):937-940

[7] Olsen RW, Sieghart W. International Union of Pharmacology. LXX. Subtypes of gamma-aminobutyric acid(A) receptors: Classification on the basis of subunit composition, pharmacology, and function. Update. Pharmacological Reviews. 2008;**60**(3):243-260

[8] Fritschy JM, Brunig I. Formation and plasticity of GABAergic synapses: Physiological mechanisms and pathophysiological implications. Pharmacology & Therapeutics. 2003; **98**(3):299-323

[9] Lin SC, Bergles DE. Synaptic signaling between neurons and glia. Glia. 2004;**47**(3):290-298

[10] Korpi ER, Grunder G, Luddens H. Drug interactions at GABA(A) receptors. Progress in Neurobiology. 2002;**67**(2):113-159

[11] Vlainić J, Jembrek MJ, Strac DS, Pericić D. The effects of zolpidem treatment and withdrawal on the in vitro expression of recombinant alpha1beta2gamma2s GABA(A) receptors expressed in HEK 293 cells. Naunyn-Schmiedeberg's Archives of Pharmacology. 2010;**382**(3):201-212

[12] Chebib M, Johnston GA. GABA-activated ligand gated ion channels: Medicinal chemistry and molecular biology. Journal of Medicinal Chemistry. 2000;**43**(8):1427-1447

[13] Bettler B, Kaupmann K, Mosbacher J, Gassmann M. Molecular structure and physiological functions of GABA(B) receptors. Physiological Reviews. 2004;**84**(3):835-867

[14] Heaney CF, Kinney JW. Role of GABA(B) receptors in learning and memory and neurological disorders. Neuroscience and Biobehavioral Reviews. 2016;**63**:1-28

[15] Cryan JF, Kaupman K. Don't worry 'B' happy!: A role for $GABA_B$ receptors in anxiety and depression. Trends in Pharmacological Sciences. 2005;**26**(1):36-43

[16] Bowery NG. $GABA_B$ receptor: A site of therapeutic benefit. Current Opinion in Pharmacology. 2006;**6**(1):37-43

[17] Meldrum BS. Glutamate as a neurotransmitter in the brain: Review of physiology and pathology. The Journal of Nutrition. 2000;**130**(4S):1007S-10015S

[18] Lesage A, Steckler T. Metabotropic glutamate mGlu1 receptor stimulation and blockade: Therapeutic opportunities in psychiatric illness. European Journal of Pharmacology. 2010;**639**(1-3):2-16

[19] Paoletti P, Neyton J. NMDA receptor subunits: Function and pharmacology. Current Opinion in Pharmacology. 2007;**7**(1):39-47

[20] Kleckner NW, Dingledine R. Requirement for glycine in activation of NMDA-receptors expressed in Xenopus oocytes. Science. 1988;**241**(4867):835-837

[21] Lee MC, Ting KK, Adams S, Brew BJ, Chung R, Guillemin GJ. Characterisation of the expression of NMDA receptors in human astrocytes. PLoS One. 2010;**5**(11):e14123

[22] Barco A, Bailey CH, Kandel ER. Common molecular mechanisms in explicit and implicit memory. Journal of Neurochemistry. 2006;**97**(6):1520-1533

[23] Chen HS, Lipton SA. The chemical biology of clinically tolerated NMDA receptor antagonists. Journal of Neurochemistry. 2006;**97**(6):1611-1626

[24] Lipton SA. Paradigm shift in neuroprotection by NMDA receptor blockade: Memantine and beyond. Nature Reviews. Drug Discovery. 2006;**5**(2):160-170

[25] Koch HJ, Szecsey A, Haen E. NMDA-antagonism (memantine): An alternative pharmacological therapeutic principle in Alzheimer's and vascular dementia. Current Pharmaceutical Design. 2004;**10**(3):253-259

[26] Song I, Huganir RL. Regulation of AMPA receptors during synaptic plasticity. Trends in Neurosciences. 2002;**25**(11):578-588

[27] Mayer ML. Glutamate receptor ion channels. Current Opinion in Neurobiology. 2005; **15**(3):282-288

[28] Greger IH, Ziff EB, Penn AC. Molecular determinants of AMPA receptor subunit assembly. Trends in Neurosciences. 2007;**30**(8):407-416

[29] Rosenmund C, Stern-Bach Y, Stevens CF. The tetrameric structure of a glutamate receptor channel. Science. 1998;**280**(5369):1596-1599

[30] Platt SR. The role of glutamate in central nervous system health and disease—A review. Veterinary Journal. 2007;**173**(2):278-286

[31] Evans AJ, Gurung S, Henley JM, Nakamura Y, Wilkinson KA. Exciting times: New advances towards understanding the regulation and roles of kainate receptors. Neurochemical Research. 2017 [Epub ahead of print]

[32] Niswender CM, Conn PJ. Metabotropic glutamate receptors: Physiology, pharmacology, and disease. Annual Review of Pharmacology and Toxicology. 2010;**50**:295-322

[33] Swanson CJ, Bures M, Johnson MP, Linden AM, Monn JA, Schoepp DD. Metabotropic glutamate receptors as novel targets for anxiety and stress disorders. Nature Reviews. Drug Discovery. 2005;**4**(2):131-144

[34] Samardzic J, Svob Strac D. Benzodiazepines and Anxiety disorders: From laboratory to clinic. In: Durbano F, editor. New Developments in Anxiety Disorders. Rijeka: InTech; 2016. pp. 23-45

[35] Jadzic D. Role of the Bed Nucleus of Stria Terminalis (BNST) in addiction and depression: a microdialysis study [PhD thesis]. University of Cagliari; 2018

[36] Car H, Wiśniewski K. Similarities and interactions between GABAergic and glutaminergic systems. Roczniki Akademii Medycznej w Białymstoku. 1998;**43**:5-26

Chapter 2

Early Life Experience, Maternal Separation, and Involvement of GABA and Glutamate Transporters

Gabriela Beatriz Acosta

Additional information is available at the end of the chapter

http://dx.doi.org/10.5772/intechopen.70868

Abstract

The physiological response initiates with activation of the hypothalamic-pituitary-adrenal axis, the autonomic nervous, and the immune systems. All actions promoted cellular adaptive changes in cells and tissues that protect the body and promote their survival. Diverse protocols of maternal separation (MS) in rodents presented alterations in central nervous system (CNS) such as learning disabilities, voluntary alcohol intake, and neurochemical changes. It is believed that the properties of these early life procedures are mediated by the high plasticity of the developing CNS. During critical development stage, brain regions, mainly those related to aggressive conditions, can have advancement abnormalities occasionally irreversible and thus adjust emotional processing when they grow to be adults. Early postnatal period and relationship between mother and infant are essential of normal stress response and emotional behavior. Probably, it involves the activation of intracellular signaling pathways, genome adaptations, adjusts in gene expression, and neural action. The objective of this article is to provide an overview of the current state of knowledge in the field focused on the maternal separation model, early life experience of postnatal stress, and the involvement of γ-aminobutyric acid (GABA) and glutamate transporters.

Keywords: development plasticity, early maternal separation, acute and chronic stress, transporters, GABA, glutamate

1. Introduction

Actually, it has been accepted that postnatal exposure to adverse events like stress can influence the offspring neurodevelopment, its neuroendocrine, and immune systems and induce behavioral changes thus disturbing neuroplasticity [1, 2].

The central nervous system (CNS) maintains a degree of adaptive plasticity, which allows adjusting to certain situations and adapting innate designs from neuronal connections. There is an abundant bibliography where it is shown that the unfavorable measures in the early life of an individual present profound and persistent effects on the cerebral functions, being able to represent a risky influence for the future development of the psychopathology [4, 5]. Epidemiological studies have shown that postnatal stress or emotional trauma, especially when suffering from early life, is usually associated with an increased possibility of depression [6]. During the critical period of certain brain regions, mainly those related to adverse situations, such as the frontal cortex (CF), hippocampus (Hic), and amygdala, hypothalamic-pituitary-adrenal (HPA) axis can develop almost irreversible abnormalities and alter the response to stress throughout the life of the animal [6, 7]. A recent study of the consequences of maltreatment and stress during childhood at early ages has shown the effects of this experience on brain structures. These structural changes were associated with changes in levels of stress hormones and neurotransmitters, resulted in maltreatment and stress in childhood at early ages, a variety of disorders including depression, anxiety, aggression, impulsivity, hyperactivity, criminal tendency, or abuse of toxic substances [8–11]. With all these evidences, we can deduce that an excess of stress at early ages of the developing life restricts with the paused, progressive, and normal development of the brain [5, 12, 13].

The brain is vulnerable to early-life programming, and this can be manifested in childhood or adulthood as stress hyper-reactivity by deregulation of the HPA axis and increased susceptibility to affective disorders like anxiety, depression, and schizophrenia [14, 15]. Exposure to early stressful adverse life events may increase vulnerability to psychopathology in adult life. There are important memory disturbances in stress-related psychiatric disorders [16].

The term neuroplasticity refers to the potential of the brain to reorganize by creating new neural pathways to adapt, as it needs [2]. This phenomenon requires the stable modulation of gene expression, which is mediated at least in part by epigenetic processes such as DNA methylation and histone modifications. Both the genome and the epigenome cooperate interactively in the mature phenotype and determine the sensitivity to environmental factors and the subsequent risk of disease [17–19]. There is increasing evidence that environmental factors, particularly stressful events experienced early in life, increase the risk of developing a psychiatric illness and/or a behavioral disorder [3, 18, 19]. The experiences of chronic stress are a factor that mainly influences numerous neuropsychiatric diseases, since it often leads to maladaptive responses [20].

While the childhood adversity as a negative childhood experience associated with increased lifetime risk of poorer health and social outcomes have been described postnatal experiences. Several studies in psychiatry have shown a long-term negative effect on health and society such as depression [21], alcohol abuse, use of consumer drugs, family abuse, and other social practices that interact with these processes [22].

The aim of this article is to overview on the current state of knowledge in the field focusing an animal model of maternal separation (MS), early life experience of postnatal stress, and the involvement of γ-aminobutyric acid (GABA) and glutamate transporters.

2. Early environmental experiences

The brain in the early stages of development presents a high level of plasticity, facilitating both adaptive variations on behalf of opportunities, and malformations alterable vulnerability. At present, neuropsychiatric illnesses evident as complex combinations of cognitive, emotional, and behavioral discrepancies have their origins of development fixed primary in the initial placement of the functional impression of the brain [23]. Postnatal periods are critical for CNS development [24]. After birth, the brain continues to grow with its total volume doubling in the first year, measured by 15% rise in the second year [25]. In particular, this increase is explained by the development of neuronal connections in gray matter (synapses and dendrites), long-range axons, and myelination; all of these are necessary for the society of circulated functional systems; regressive development includes the pruning of the synapses and axons during the childhood period, permitting the restructuring of the primarily practical circuits [26].

Animal models are useful tools that help us to understand how genetic vulnerability factors can modulate responses to early environmental factors and provide insights into behavioral and physiological mechanisms involved in the pathways through which early stress might produce long-term effects. In this review, we will focus in the models of MS.

3. Maternal separation

Adverse childhood experience is considered one of the main risk factors for the development of psychopathology. Maternal separation in rodents (rats or mice) is a well-known animal model of early stress to explore the neuroendocrine and behavioral properties of early difficulty. This paradigm discusses to the daily separation of puppies (usually rodents) from their mothers for a short period of time (1 hour) or prolonged (3–6 hours) during the first 1–3 weeks after birth. The paradigmatic MS puppies remain together as a litter [27]. This process is performed between birth and weaning for diverse periods of time and permits a set of experimental designs, which vary in the frequency, the duration, and the age at which the MS occurred.

Studies in animal models show the influence of life conditions during the postnatal period in the establishment of neurological factors that control behavior and response to stress [28]. Acute and chronic MS has both short and long-term effects on behavior and neuroendocrinal responses [29].

Different experimental protocols of MS in rodents have shown changes in CNS functioning: learning impediments, voluntary alcohol consumption, and behavioral variations [30]. This handling in animals is used for diverse experiments, for example, Studies in life sciences sometimes require repeated manipulation in rodents during the course of the experiment (handling). The main function of the handling is to minimize the stress associated with behavioral, pharmacological and endocrine studies [31–33].

The early life of most mammals is expended in near contact with the mother and for the newborn. Early MS is a traumatic occurrence that, conditioning on the different situations, can form its behavioral and neurochemical phenotype in adulthood. Studies in rodents exhibited that a very short separation cooled by a greater maternal care can completely affect the development of offspring. Nevertheless, prolonged MS origins stress. The significance of this stress and HPA axis hyper-reactivity is articulated in adulthood and continues throughout the life [34]. MS in rodents, particularly in rats, was used as a model for various psychotic conditions, especially depression and anxiety [30, 32]. The most popular MS technique of a daily separation of 3 hours from the second to the 12th postpartum day produces a model of high-construct depression and predictive validity. The results of studies of MS in rat lead to a discussion to its benefits for the neonates. This procedure might be contributed for the mental health of the offspring in adulthood [34].

4. Physiological mechanisms involved in early maternal separation: neurobiological responses to early life stress

4.1. HPA axis

The hypothalamo-pituitary-adrenal axis is a key component of the stress reaction. Many studies have shown the impact of stress exposure during development on the HPA axis activity and on psychoemotional disorders during adulthood [19, 35].

Lifelong variations in HPA axis perform examined as a result of developmental complexities (maternal separation) demonstrate connections with psychiatric disorders containing schizophrenia depression, which may be characterized by irregularities in the activity of HPA axis and reaction to stress [4, 36, 37].

4.2. Neurotrophins reaction

Neurotrophins, also called neurotrophic factors, are a family of proteins that favor the survival of neurons. Family members include nerve growth factor (NGF), brain-derived neurotrophic factor (BDNF), neurotrophin-3 (NT-3), and neurotrophin 4/5 (NT4/5) [38–40]. During development, limiting amounts of neurotrophins function as survival factors to ensure a match between the number of surviving neurons and the requirement for appropriate target innervation. In addition, they arrange cell destiny decisions, axon growth, dendrite pruning, the pattern of innervation, and the expression of proteins critical for normal neuronal role, such as neurotransmitters and ion channels. In the adult CNS, they control synaptic activity and plasticity, while ongoing to modulate neuronal survival [41].

4.3. Neurochemical response

Adverse early life practices can provoke neurochemical alterations that may underlie modifications in HPA axis reaction, emotionality, and cognition [42]. The impact of stress on brain function is known. Different substances are released in response to stress and can influence various neural circuits. The individual effects of functional neuronal mediators of stress (neurotransmitters, neuropeptides, and steroids) and plasticity are integrated. This causes the stress instruments to produce an orchestrated “symphony” that allows for adjusted responses to the various challenges [42]. Different neurotransmitters, such as NA, 5-HT, Glutamate, and

GABA, and neuromodulators, such as neuropeptide Y, oxytocin, a gaseous molecule, and nitric oxide, have been implicated in the pathogenesis of stress-dependent disorders in early stages of life [43].

We will focus on the GABA and Glutamate neurotransmission, especially in their transporters.

5. γ-Aminobutyric acid (GABA)

γ-aminobutyric acid (GABA) is the chief inhibitory neurotransmitter of the adult mammalian CNS. During the early post-natal development, GABA acts as an excitatory neurotransmitter, serving as a neuronal and neurotrophic migration factor, separately from taking part in synaptogenesis. The GABAergic system has a large, complete molecular machine, by which it performs its actions, including enzymes for its synthesis and metabolism, membrane receptors, and transport proteins. Recent literature demonstrates that GABA transporters, as well as the GABAA receptor, are proteins of importance for the normal functioning and development of the central nervous system. All these molecules allow GABA to perform an essential function, both in the developing brain as in the adult brain. For this reason, the expression profile of the different subtypes of the molecules previously mentioned will be described in this article, in order to obtain a thorough knowledge of the molecular behavior of the GABAergic system from conception to adulthood [44, 45].

During the early postnatal development, GABA acts as an excitatory neurotransmitter, serving as a neuronal and neurotrophic migration factor, apart from taking part in synaptogenesis. The GABAergic system has a large, complete molecular machine, by which it performs its actions, including enzymes for its synthesis and metabolism, membrane receptors, and transport proteins. There is abundant literature showing that GABA transporters, as well as the GABA A receptor, are proteins of particular importance for the normal functioning and development of the central nervous system [46–49]. GABA-mediated inhibition exerts a powerful control over cortical neuronal activity, and GABA transporters (GATs) contribute to modulate the action of GABA [45]. Altered GATs activity and/or expression are likely to affect markedly cortical function, with their possible involvement in the pathophysiology of selected human disease.

5.1. Transporters of GABA (GATs)

The regulation of extracellular levels of GABA is essential for normal CNS development and functioning. The principal mechanism by which the levels of the neurotransmitter are regulated is through Na^+-dependent high-affinity uptake carried out by synaptic and glial located transporter proteins called GABA transporters [50]. The others GAT-1, GAT-2, and GAT-3 have been identified from the GATs identified and cloned, although there is also a fourth isoform, BGT-1 (Betaine Carrier/GABA). Although all these transporter molecules have high affinity and selectivity for GABA, they present differential characteristics in pharmacology, localization, and functionality [13, 50, 51]. In fact, the levels of expression during postnatal CNS development vary markedly between the two transporters [13, 52]. There is another GAT, located intracellularly, which is the vesicular GABA transporter (VGAT), which plays a primordial role in the normal development of the immature brain [52].

- **GAT-1**: This transporter is one of the most important isoforms of GATs. They are brain-specific proteins [53–56]. This transporter has the particularity of being found in both neurons and glial cells and is the main isoform of GATs in the mature brain [52].

- **GAT-2**: It is the least abundant isoform. Although low levels of GAT-2 have been detected in GABAergic neurons, this transporter is considered as extraparenchymal and its localization is limited to leptomeningeal and ependymal cells [52, 57]. In all postnatal stages, GAT-2 is detected in the arachnoid layer and in the arachnoid trabecula of the subarachnoid space. In some cases, expression of GAT-2 is observed across the entire diameter of the blood vessels supplying the cortex. The latter characteristic occurs mainly between postnatal day 0 and 5, and this transporter may be considered as the main source of peripheral GABA [52].

- **GAT-3**: This isoform of the GABA transporter is among the most abundant along with GAT-1. GAT-3 is the predominant isoform during the early postnatal stages regulating neuronal excitability at these times [52, 58] and has its unique location in astrocytes [52].

- **VGAT**: The vesicular GABA transporter is essential for GABAergic neurotransmission to occur, as it introduces GABA into the presynaptic vesicles using a proton gradient. In this way, the GABA is stored to be released after the arrival of an action potential to the presynaptic terminal [59].

Odeon et al. [60] evaluated the effects of acute MS (AMS) and CMS (Chronic MS) + cold stress on the expression levels of GAT-1 in FC and Hic, whose appearance correlates with the concentration of corticosterone at different postnatal day from birth to young adulthood. In response to AMS + cold stress in FC, they demonstrated a decrease expression of GAT-1 at PD13. But in CMS, the levels of GAT-1 increased both at PD57 and PD63. At AMS in HIc, they observed an enhance in GAT-1 expression of either PD7 or PD13. Conversely, CMS decreased either PD57 or PD67 and increased at PD71 hippocampal levels expression of GAT-1. With respect to the levels of corticosterone, they observed an increase in all age groups studied in AMS. On the contrary, they showed a decrease in corticosterone levels in CMS. These authors concluded that a low responsiveness of the early postnatal period to stress, involvement of GABAergic system, suggesting that GATs may contribute to the deregulation of neuronal excitability that accompanies at neurobiological consequences of early stress. These dates obtained in this experimental condition serve as a starting point, elucidating the molecular mechanism of GAT regulation in GABA system throughout postnatal development.

In homogenates of FC and Hic acquired from either acute or chronic MS + cold stress, we found variations on the expression of GAT-1. GABA system plays a role in the pathophysiology of anxiety and mood disorders. The extracellular levels of GABA are regulated by specific high-affinity transporters, one of which, the plasma membrane GAT1, is considered the predominant neuronal transporter in the rodent brain [56, 61].

Although AMS might mimic a "dramatic" experience occurring at a precise developmental stage, the less dramatic repeated maternal separation can reproduce a more physiological situation [6].

The central nervous system maintains a degree of adaptive plasticity, which allows it to adjust to certain conditions and modify the innate patterns of neuronal connections [62]. These mediators exert a paradoxical damage-protection action. These variations can alter the functioning of the CNS, and consequently, the body's response to stress throughout life, as this treatment is done during the postnatal period, with the CNS in full development. A further support to this possibility came from the demonstration that prepulse inhibition disruption in maternally deprived rats occurs only after puberty [63, 64], with a temporal profile similar to the onset of schizophrenic symptomatology in patients, and was reversed by treatment with typical and atypical antipsychotic drugs [34], suggesting that the defects resulting from MS might be the consequence of an hyperactivity of the dopaminergic system [65].

The identification of neurobiological substrates that are affected by early life adverse experience may have important diagnostic implications and could contribute to identify novel molecular targets for the development of more effective treatments of psychiatric disorders. Further studies are now warranted to elucidate the type or the timing of early life events that are associated with enhanced risk for depression or anxiety may be different from those relevant to schizophrenia [66].

6. Glutamate

We will briefly describe glutamate as the main excitatory neurotransmitter in the brain. There are three families of ionotropic receptors with channels permeable to intrinsic cations: N-methyl-D-aspartate (NMDA), α- amino-3-hydroxy-5-methyl-4-isoxazolpropionic acid (AMPA), and Kainate. There are three groups of metabotropics, protein G-coupled glutamate receptors (mGluR) that modify neuronal and glial excitability through G-protein subunits acting on membrane ion channels and second messengers such as diacylglycerol and cAMP. Endogenous glutamate, by activating NMDA, AMPA or mGluR1 receptors, may contribute to acute brain damage following epilepsy, cerebral ischemia, or traumatic brain injury. It may also contribute to chronic neurodegeneration in disorders such as amyotrophic lateral sclerosis and Huntington's chorea. In animal models of cerebral ischemia and traumatic brain injury, NMDA and AMPA receptor antagonists protect against acute brain damage and delayed behavioral deficits. Other clinical conditions including epilepsy, amnesia, anxiety, and psychosis may respond to drugs that act on glutamatergic transmission [67, 68].

6.1. Transporters of glutamate (GluTs)

A family of transporter proteins, excitatory amino acid transporters (EAAT), regulates extracellular concentration of Glu. Several lines of evidence suggest that increases of Glu in extracellular levels are involved in the stress response [68]. Astrocytes are the main protectors of neurons from excitotoxicity in the normal CNS, and this protection is conferred by clearance of extracellular [69].

The GluTs family is mediated by Na + dependent high affinity, this represents a critical factor in the Glu uptake and the regulation of homeostasis in the synaptic cleft [70]. Five high-affinity GluTs were cloned into human and animal tissues and identified as a glutamate aspartate transporter (GLAST), excitatory amino acid carrier-1 (EAAT)-1, glial glutamate transporter-1 (GLT-1, EAAT-2); excitatory amino acid-carrier-1 (EAAC-1, EAAT-3), EAAT-4, and EAAT-5. Unlike other neurotransmitters, the action of Glu released into the synaptic cleft is terminated by uptake into neurons and surrounding glial cells via specific transporters. Within the nerve terminal, the glutamine released by glial cells and taken up by neurons is converted back to Glu [71]. Rapid removal of Glu from the extracellular space is required for the survival and normal function of neurons. Although GluTs are expressed by all CNS cell types, astrocytes are the cell type primarily responsible for Glu uptake [72]. Astrocytes express both GLT-1 and GLAST, while axon terminals in the neocortex only express GLT-1.

Previous studies have indicated that exposure to variable types of stressors during development produces persistent behavioral defects that are associated with hormonal, neurotransmitters, transporters, and functional changes, and resemble an array of psychopathological conditions.

Altered glutamate receptor (GluR) expression has been implicated in the pathogenesis of stress-induced disorders. Adrover et al. [73] have shown that glutamate neurotransmission might be impaired in the brain of prenatally stressed rats. They observed an increased uptake capacity for glutamate in the PFC of prenatal stress males, while no such changes were observed in the Hic. They concluded that prenatal stress produced long-term changes in the glutamatergic system, modulating the expression of glutamate transporters and altering synaptic transmission in the adult brain.

Odeon et al. [74] found that both ethanol intake and activity and protein expression of GluTs in certain areas of the rat brain are affected by repeated maternal separation (RMS). Also, they demonstrated that RMS increases glutamate uptake in frontal cortex and hippocampus, and RMS reduced both GLT-1 and EAAT-3 protein expression and increased GLAST protein levels.

Social loneliness has been used intensively as an animal model to study the consequences of social isolation during childhood on the brain and behavior. There is a crucial stage during which social isolation has very profound and sometimes irreversible effects.

Recent studies indicate that there are many aspects of alcohol and drug dependence that involve changes in glutamate transmission. Different investigations have reported that drugs of abuse, including alcohol and cocaine, modify GluTs [75, 76]. The effects of ethanol on glutamate transport may be mediated in part by the level of Ca^{2+}/calmodulin kinase activity [77]. Similarly, Othman et al. [78] indicated that in rat cortical astrocytes *in vitro* ethanol affects [^{3}H]-Glutamate uptake by affecting protein kinase C (PKC) modulation of transporter activity.

Odeon et al. [74] observed changes following RMS in the glutamatergic system which could be an effect of glucocorticoid. It is known that this hormone may regulate GluT expression [79] and ethanol intake [80]. A significant increase in glutamate uptake is observed. However, protein levels of the major glial (GLT-1) and neuronal (EAAT-3) transporters declined. It should be noted that a third glutamate transporter, GLAST, was found in glia of the frontal cortex, and hippocampus was studied. This transporter exhibits increased levels of protein expression after treatment. This could be due to the decreased expression of the major glutamate uptake proteins and the probable excitotoxic consequence, which triggered a compensatory mechanism through the increase of GLAST.

GluTs are neuronal and non-neuronal factors necessary for expression, maintenance, and transcriptional regulators of these proteins. The finding that RMS altered Glu regulation in the frontal cortex and hippocampus indicates a possible role for distorted glutamate regulation in the causal relationship between early life stress. Finally, I have some specific questions about this work: (1) Can early exposures with limited time produce lasting physiological changes? (2) Can these physiological changes lead to illness? (3) What factors could induce susceptibility to the adversity of normal development? Responses to these questions should influence the awareness of all social areas for the child's well-being and health throughout life.

7. Conclusions

The findings reviewed here explore some biological mechanisms that could explain the linkages between childhood negative experiences, possible diseases, and function of glutamate and GABA transporters. These results demonstrate efforts to improve quality of life throughout life. With the emergence of new tools, such as the biomarkers of early adversity, this will enable a new path of research with the close collaboration of physicians, health professionals, families, and communities on the basis of a deep understanding of the long term from early adversity.

Acknowledgements

This work was supported by UBACYT grants B019 from the University of Buenos Aires and PIP N° 114-2009-0100118 from National Scientific and Technologic Research Council (CONICET) to GBA. GBA is member of CONICET.

Conflict of interest

The authors report no conflicts of interest. The authors alone are responsible for the content and writing of the paper.

Author details

Gabriela Beatriz Acosta

Address all correspondence to: gacosta@ffyb.uba.ar

Institute of Pharmacological Research (ININFA), National Scientific and Technologic Research Council (CONICET), School of Pharmacy and Biochemistry, University of Buenos Aires, Buenos Aires, Argentina

References

[1] McEwen BS, Gianaros PJ. Stress-and allostasis-induced brain plasticity. Annual Review of Medicine. 2011;**62**:431-445

[2] Deppermann S, Storchak H, Fallgatter AJ, Ehlis A-C. Stress-induced neuroplasticity: (Mal) adaptation to adverse life events in patients with PTSD. A critical overview. Neuroscience. 2014;**283**:166-177

[3] Odeon MM, Salatino AE, Acosta GB. Consequences of postnatal stress: Maternal separation in rats induces long-lasting changes on glutamate transporters. Clinical and Experimental Pharmacology. 2013;**3**(2):121-125

[4] Arborelius L, Owens MJ, Plotsky PM, Nemeroff CB. The role of corticotropin-releasing factor in depression and anxiety disorders. The Journal of Endocrinology. 1999;**160**:1-12

[5] Smith SM, Vale WW. The role of the hypothalamic-pituitary-adrenal axis in neuroendocrine responses to stress. Dialogues in Clinical Neuroscience. 2006;**8**:383-395

[6] Fumagalli F, Molteni R, Racagni G, Riva MA. Stress during development: Impact on neuroplasticity and relevance to psychopathology. Progress in Neurobiology. 2007;**1**(4):197-217

[7] Pryce CR, Rüedi-Bettschen D, Dettling AC, Weston A, Russig H, Ferger B, Feldon J. Long-term effects of early-life environmental manipulations in rodents and primates: Potential animal in depression research. Neuroscience and Biobehavioral Reviews. 2005;**29**:649-674

[8] Maccari S, Krugers HJ, Morley-Fletcher S, Szyf M, Brunton PJ. The consequences of early-life adversity: Neurobiological: Behavioural and epigenetic adaptations. Journal of Neuroendocrinology. 2014;**26**:707-723

[9] Fletcher A, Bonell C, Hargreaves J. School effects on young people's drug use: A systematic review of intervention and observational studies. The Journal of Adolescent Health. 2008;**42**(3):209-220

[10] Diz-Chaves Y, Astiz M, Bellini MJ, Garcia-Segura LM. Prenatal stress increases the expression of proinflammatory cytokines and exacerbates theinflammatory response to LPS in the hippocampal formation of adult male mice. Brain, Behavior, and Immunity. 2013;**28**:196-206

[11] Berens AE, Jensen SKG, Nelson CA III. Biological embedding of childhood adversity: From physiological mechanisms to clinical implications. BMC Medicine. 2017;**15**:135-138

[12] Koenig JI, Kirkpatrick B, Lee P. Glucocorticoid hormones and early brain development in schizophrenia. Neuropsychopharmacology. 2002;**27**:309-318

[13] Lupien SJ, McEwen BS, Gunnar MR, Heim C. Effects of stress throughout the lifespan on the brain, behaviour and cognition. Nature Reviews. Neuroscience. 2009;**10**(6):434-445

[14] Kofman O. The role of prenatal stress in the etiology of developmental behavioural disorders. Neuroscience and Biobehavioral Reviews. 2002;**26**:457-470

[15] Nestler EJ. From neurobiology to treatment: Progress against addiction. Nature Neuroscience. 2002;**5**(Suppl):1076-1079

[16] Ehlert U, Gaab J, Heinrichs M. Psychoneuroendocrinological contributions to the etiology of depression, posttraumatic stress disorder, and stress-related bodily disorders: The role of the hypothalamus-pituitary-adrenal axis. Biological Psychology. 2001;**57**(1-3):141-152

[17] Gluckman PD, Hanson MA, Cooper C, Thornburg KL. Effect of in utero and early-life conditions on adult health and disease. The New England Journal of Medicine. 2008;**359**(1):61-73

[18] Zhang TY, Meaney MJ. Epigenetics and the environmental regulation of the genome and its function. Annual Review of Psychology. 2010;**61**:439-466

[19] Heim C, Plotsky PM, Nemeroff CM. Importance of studying the contributions of early adverse experience to neurobiological findings in depression. Neuropsychopharmacology. 2004;**29**:641-648

[20] Novais A, Monteiro S, Roque S, Correia-Neves M, Sousa N. How age, sex and genotype shape the stress response. Neurobiology of Stress. 2016;**6**:44-45

[21] Bellis MA, Lowey H, Leckenby N, Hughes K, Harrison D. Adverse childhood experiences: Retrospective study to determine the impact on adult health behaviours and health outcomes in a UK population. Journal of Public Health (Oxford). 2014;**36**:81-91

[22] Beckie TM. A systematic review of allostatic load, health, and health disparities. Biological Research for Nursing. 2012;**14**:311-346

[23] Beardslee WR, Chien PL, Bell CC. Prevention of mental disorders, substance abuse, and problem behaviors: A developmental perspective. Psychiatric Services. 2011;**62**:247-254

[24] Ismail FY, Fatemi A, Johnston MV. Cerebral plasticity: Windows of opportunity in the developing brain. European Journal of Paediatric Neurology. 2017;**21**(1):23-48

[25] Knickmeyer RC, Gouttard S, Kang C, Evans D, Wilber K, Smith JK, Hamer RM, Lin W, Gerig G, Gilmore JH. A structural MRI study of human brain development from birth to 2 years. The Journal of Neuroscience. 2008;**28**:12176-12182

[26] Levitt P. Structural and functional maturation of the developing primate brain. The Journal of Pediatrics. 2003;**143**:S35-S45

[27] Lehmann J, Feldon J. Long-term biobehavioral effects of maternal separation in the rat: Consistent or confusing? Reviews in the Neurosciences. 2000;**11**(4):383-408

[28] Marco EM, Adriani W, Llorente R, Laviola G, Viveros MP. Detrimental psychophysiological effects of early maternal deprivation in adolescent and adult rodents: Altered responses to cannabinoid exposure. Neuroscience and Biobehavioral Reviews. 2009;**33**:498-507

[29] Anisman H, Zaharia MD, Meaney MJ, Merali Z. Do early life events permanently alter behavioral and hormonal response to stressors? Int J Dev Neurosc. 1998;**16**:149-167

[30] Roman E, Gustafsson L, Berg M, Nylander I. Behavioral profiles and stress induced corticosteroid secretion in male Wistar rats subjected to short and prolonged periods of maternal separation. Hormones and Behavior. 2006;**50**:736-747

[31] O'Shea RD. Roles and regulation of glutamate transporters in the central nervous system. Clinical and Experimental Pharmacology & Physiology. 2002;**29**:1018-1023

[32] Yehuda R, Antelman SM. Criteria for rationally evaluating animal models of posttraumatic stress disorder. Biological Psychiatry. 1993;**33**:479-486

[33] Tamaki K, Yamada K, Nakamichi N, Taniura H, Yoneda Y. Transient suppression of progenitor cell proliferation through NMDA receptors in hippocampal dentate gyrus of mice with traumatic stress experience. Journal of Neurochemistry. 2008;**105**:1642-1655

[34] Kuhn CM, Pauk J, Schanberg SM. Endocrine responses to mother-infant separation in developing rats. Developmental Psychobiology. 1990;**23**:395-410

[35] Vetulani J. Early maternal separation: A rodent model of depression and a prevailing human condition. Pharmacological Reports. 2013;**65**:1451-1461

[36] Jahng JW. An animal model of eating disorders associated with stressful experience in early life. Hormones and Behavior. 2011;**59**(2):213-220

[37] Lohof AM, Ip NY, Poo MM. Potentiation of developing neuromuscular synapses by the neurotrophins NT-3 and BDNF. Nature. 1993;**363**:350-352

[38] Corcoran C, Walker E, Huot R, Mittal V, Tessner K, Kestler L, Malaspina D. The stress cascade and schizophrenia: Etiology and onset. Schizophrenia Bulletin. 2003;**29**(4):671-692

[39] de Kloet ER, Joëls M, Holsboer F. Stress and the brain: From adaptation to disease. Nature Reviews. Neuroscience 2005; **6**(6):463-475

[40] Levine ES, Dreyfus CF, Black IB, Plummer MR. Brain-derived neurotrophic factor rapidly enhances synaptic transmission in hippocampal neurons via postsynaptic tyrosine kinase receptors. Proceedings of the National Academy of Sciences of the United States of America. 1995;**92**:8074-8077

[41] Huang EJ, Reichardt LF. Neurotrophins: Roles in neuronal development and function. Annual Review of Neuroscience. 2001;**24**:677-736

[42] Giachino C, Canalia N, Capone F, Fasolo A, Alleva E, Riva MA, Cirulli F, Peretto P. Maternal deprivation and early handling affect density of calcium binding protein-containing neurons in selected brain regions and emotional behavior in periadolescent rats. Neuroscience. 2007;**145**(2):568-578

[43] Joëls M, Baram TZ. The neuro-symphony of stress. Nature Reviews. Neuroscience. 2009; **10**(6):459-466

[44] Borden LA. GABA transporter heterogeneity: Pharmacology and cellular localization. Neurochemistry International. 1996;(4):335-356

[45] Conti F, Minelli A, Melone M. GABA transporters in the mammalian cerebral cortex: Localization, development and pathological implications. Brain Research Brain Research Review. 2004;**3**:196-212

[46] Ganguly K, Schinder AF, Wong ST, Poo M. GABA itself promotes the developmental switch of neuronal GABAergic responses from excitation to inhibition. Cell. 2001;**105**(4):521-532

[47] Ben-Ari Y. Excitatory actions of GABA during development: The nature of the nurture. Nature Reviews. Neuroscience. 2002;(9):728-739

[48] Tyzio R, Minlebaev M, Rheims S, Ivanov A, Jorquera I, Holmes GL, Zilberter Y, Ben-Ari Y, Khazipov R. Postnatal changes in somatic gamma-aminobutyric acid signalling in the rat hippocampus. The European Journal of Neuroscience. 2008;**27**(10):2515-2528

[49] Yamada J, Okabe A, Toyoda H, Kilb W, Luhmann HJ, Fukuda A. Cl- uptake promoting depolarizing GABA actions in immature rat neocortical neurones is mediated by NKCC1. The Journal of Physiology. 2004;**557**(Pt 3):829-841

[50] McEwen BS. Sex, stress and the hippocampus: Allostasis, allostatic load and the aging process. Neurobiology of Aging. 2002;**23**(5):921-939

[51] McEwen BS. Physiology and neurobiology of stress and adaptation: Central role of the brain. Physiological Reviews. 20071;**87**(3):873-904

[52] Minelli A, Barbaresi P, Conti F. Postnatal development of high-affinity plasma membrane GABA transporters GAT-2 and GAT-3 in the rat cerebral cortex. Brain Research. Developmental Brain Research. 2003;**142**(1):7-18

[53] Yan XX, Cariaga WA, Ribak CE. Immunoreactivity for GABA plasma membrane transporter, GAT-1, in the developing rat cerebral cortex: Transient presence in the somata of neocortical and hippocampal neurons. Brain Research. Developmental Brain Research. 1997;**99**(1):1-19

[54] Ikegaki N, Saito N, Hashima M, Tanaka C. Production of specific antibodies against GABA transporter subtypes (GAT-1, GAT-2, GAT-3) and their application to immunocytochemistry. Molecular Brain Research. 1994;**26**:47-54

[55] Liu QR, Lopez-Caarcuera B, Mandiyan S, Nelson H, Nelson N. Molecular characterization of four pharmacological distinct γ -aminobutyric acid transporters in the mouse brain. The Journal of Biological Chemistry. 1993;**268**(3):2106-2112

[56] Radian R, Ottersen OP, Storm-Mathisen J, Castel M, Kanner BI. Immunocytochemical localization of the GABA transporter in rat brain. The Journal of Neuroscience. 1990;**10**(4): 1319-1330

[57] Conti F, Vitellaro-Zuccarello L, Barbaresi P, Minelli A, Brecha NCMelone M. Neuronal, glial, and epithelial localization of γ -aminobutyric acid transporter 2, a high-affinity γ -aminobutyric acid plasma membrane transporter, in the cerebral cortex and neighboring structures. The Journal of Comparative Neurology. 1999;**409**(3):482-494

[58] Kinney GA. GAT-3 transporters regulate inhibition in the neocortex. Journal of Neurophysiology. 2005;**94**(6):4533-4537

[59] Minelli A, Alonso-Nanclares L, Edwards RH, De Felipe J, Conti F. Postnatal development of the vesicular GABA transporter in rat cerebral cortex. Neuroscience. 2003;**117**(2): 337-346

[60] Odeon MM, Salatino AE, Acosta GB. Consequences of early adverse life events on GABAergic neurons produce long term changes in brain function. Trends in Comparative Biochemistry & Physiology. 2011;**15**:67-72

[61] Perego C, Bulbarelli A, Longhi R, Caimi M, Villa A, Caplan MJ, Pietrini G. Sorting of two polytopic proteins, the gamma-aminobutyric acid and betaine transporters, in polarized epithelial cells. The Journal of Biological Chemistry. 1997;**272**(10):6584-6592

[62] Levine S, Mody T. The long-term psychobiological consequences of intermittent post-natal separation in the squirrel monkey. Neuroscience and Biobehavioral Reviews. 2003;**27**(1-2):83-89

[63] Ellenbroek BA, van den Kroonenberg PT, Cools AR. The effects of an early stressful life event on sensorimotor gating in adult rats. Schizophrenia Research 1998;**30**(3):251-260

[64] Lehmann J, Stöhr T, Schuller J, Domeney A, Heidbreder C, Feldon J. Long-term effects of repeated maternal separation on three different latent inhibition paradigms. Pharmacology, Biochemistry, and Behavior. 1998;**59**(4):873-882

[65] Ellenbroek BA, Cools AR. The long-term effects of maternal deprivation depend on the genetic background. Neuropsychopharmacology. 2000;**23**(1):99-106

[66] Komuro H, Rakic P. Modulation of neuronal migration by NMDA receptors. Science. 1993;**260**:95-97

[67] LoTurco JJ, Blanton MG, Kriegstein AR. Initial expression and endogenous activation of NMDA channels in early neocortical development. The Journal of Neuroscience. 1991; **11**:792-799

[68] Reznikov LR, Grillo CA, Piroli GG, Pasumarthi RK, Reagan LP, Fadel J. Acute stress-mediated increases in extracellular glutamate levels in the rat amygdala: Differential effects of antidepressant treatment. The European Journal of Neuroscience. 2007;**25**(10): 3109-3114

[69] Matute C, Alberdi E, Ibarretxe G, Sánchez-Gómez MV. Excitotoxicity in glial cells. European Journal of Pharmacology. 2002;**447**(2-3):239-246

[70] Thomas CG, Tian H, Diamond JS. The relative roles of diffusion and uptake in clearing synaptically released glutamate change during early postnatal development. The Journal of Neuroscience. 2011;**31**(12):4743-4754

[71] Kanai Y, Smith CP, Hediger MA. The elusive transporters with a high affinity for glutamate. Trends in Neurosciences. 1993;(9):365-370

[72] Anderson CM, Swanson RA. Astrocyte glutamate transport: Review of properties, regulation, and physiological functions. Glia. 2000, 2000;**32**(1):1-14

[73] Adrover E, Pallarés ME, Baier CJ, Monteleone MC, Giuliani FA, Waagepetersen HS, Brocco MA, Cabrera R, Sonnewald U, Schousboe A, Antonelli MC. Glutamate neurotransmission is affected in prenatally stressed offspring. Neurochemistry International. 2005;**88**:73-87

[74] Odeon MM, Andreu M, Yamauchi L, Grosman M, Acosta GB. Chronic postnatal stress induces voluntary alcohol intake and modifies glutamate transporters in adolescent rats. Stress. 2015;**18**(4):427-434

[75] Chappell AM, Carter E, McCool BA, Weiner JL. Adolescent rearing conditions influence the relationship between initial anxiety-like behavior and ethanol drinking in male long Evans rats. Alcoholism, Clinical and Experimental Research. 2013;**37**(Suppl 1):E394-E403

[76] Rao PSS, Sari Y. Glutamate transporter 1: Target for the treatment of alcohol dependence. Current Medicinal Chemistry. 2012;**19**:5148-5156

[77] Smith TL, Navratilova E. Increased calcium/calmodulin protein kinase activity in astrocytes chronically exposed to ethanol: Influences on glutamate transport. Neuroscience Letters. 1999;**269**(3):145-148

[78] Othman T, Sinclair CJ, Haughey N, Geiger JD, Parkinson FE. Ethanol alters glutamate but not adenosine uptake in rat astrocytes: Evidence for protein kinase C involvement. Neurochemical Research. 2002;**27**(4):289-296

[79] Danbolt NC. Glutamate uptake. Progress in Neurobiology. 2001;**65**(1):1-105

[80] Costin BN, Wolen AR, Fitting S, Shelton KL, Miles MF. Role of adrenal glucocorticoid-signaling in prefrontal cortex gene expression and acute behavioral responses to ethanol. Alcoholism, Clinical and Experimental Research. 2013;**37**(1):57-66

Chapter 3

Notch Signaling in the Astroglial Phenotype: Relevance to Glutamatergic Transmission

López-Bayghen Esther, Angulo-Rojo Carla,
López-Bayghen Bruno,
Hernández-Melchor Dinorah, Ramírez Leticia and
Ortega Arturo

Additional information is available at the end of the chapter

http://dx.doi.org/10.5772/intechopen.73318

Abstract

Glutamate (Glu), the major excitatory neurotransmitter, elicits its action through the activation of membrane receptors and transporters expressed in neurons and glial cells. Glial glutamate transporters, EAAT1 and EAAT2, remove this transmitter from the synaptic cleft preventing an excitotoxic insult. The Notch pathway is a signaling system involved in neuro- and gliogenesis. Radial glia (RG) generates neurons, oligodendrocytes, and astrocytes in a spatial and temporal pattern, in which Notch represses neurogenesis, maintaining the self-renewal potential of RG. Astrogenesis depends on several stimuli, Notch being a master regulator of the differentiation process. The cAMP-PKA-CREB signaling cascade cross talks with the Notch pathway, acting synergistically by reducing progenitor markers and inducing astrocytic differentiation. Notch1 mRNA is upregulated in a PKA/γ-secretase/NICD/CSL-dependent manner, suggesting a feedback loop to keep Notch active until astrocytic differentiation is complete. Glial differentiation is also modulated by PKC, which acts over NICD. In RG cells and astrocytes enwrapping glutamatergic synapses, EAAT1 transcriptional regulation is mediated by PKC, increasing Notch expression and its receptor intracellular traffic. It is clear that Notch represents an activity-dependent molecular key in RG cells that enable them to shape glutamatergic transmission through the expression of genes involved in glial/neuronal interactions.

Keywords: glia cells, signal transduction, Notch, differentiation, protein kinase C

1. Introduction

Glutamate (Glu), the major excitatory neurotransmitter in the central nervous system (CNS), is a key player in higher brain functions such as learning and memory, and it is also involved in cell differentiation and synaptogenesis. Glu exerts its function through specific receptors, according to which the signal transduction pathway mechanisms are classified into two major groups: ionotropic (iGluRs) and metabotropic receptors (mGluRs). iGluRs are ligand-gated ion channels subdivided upon pharmacological and electrophysiological properties into NMDA, AMPA, and KA receptors. mGluRs are G protein-coupled receptors subdivided in accordance with their amino acidic sequence and pharmacological properties into three subgroups, preferentially activated by quisqualate (Quis), t-ACPD, and L-AP4, respectively [1–4].

Cerebellar Bergmann glia cells (BGC) are radial glia (RG) cells that are not differentiated into astrocytes after birth [5] and function as a neuronal reservoir [6, 7]. These cells extend processes through the molecular layer completely surrounding excitatory synapses between Purkinje cells and both parallel and climbing fibers. An exquisite and complex interplay between presynaptic-postsynaptic neurons and glia cells is fundamental for glutamatergic transmission. Glu recycling depends upon these interactions. Glu is removed from the synaptic cleft by a family of electrogenic sodium-dependent transporters expressed in neurons and glia cells [8]. Five subtypes of transporters named excitatory amino acid transporters 1-5 (EAAT1-5) have been characterized. The glial transporters EAAT-1 (GLAST) and EAAT-2 (GLT-1) account for more than 80% of the Glu uptake activity in the brain [9, 10]. Within BGC, EAAT-1/GLAST is the predominant transporter [11].

Once internalized, Glu is metabolized to Gln via Gln synthetase and released in the vicinity of the presynaptic neuron through sodium-dependent neutral amino acid transporter (SNAT) 3. Gln is then taken up by the presynaptic neuron through SNAT 2 and converted back to Glu by the enzyme glutaminase to be packed into synaptic vesicles completing the so-called Glu/Gln shuttle (reviewed in [12]). It is this kind of glial/neuronal interactions that gave rise to what has been known in the last years as a tripartite synapse [13]. Evidence suggests that Glu transporters might also participate in the signaling transactions triggered by this excitatory amino acid. In fact, Glu regulates the uptake process in a receptor-independent manner [14]. More recently, it has also been reported that EAAT-1 is coupled to the Na^{+}/K^{+} ATPase [15, 16] and to the Gln transporter SNAT3 [17].

In this context, we reviewed in this contribution the role of Notch signaling in RG focusing in its role in EAAT-1/GLAST regulation as a key element in the molecular mechanisms that support the proven glia contribution to glutamatergic neurotransmission.

2. Glutamatergic transmission: role of glial cells

Glutamate (Glu) is the major excitatory neurotransmitter in the vertebrate brain. It elicits its action through the activation of specific membrane receptors and transporters expressed both in neurons and in glial cells. Extracellular glutamate levels have to be tightly regulated in order to prevent Glu receptors over-stimulation that has been shown to result in neuronal death, phenomena commonly known as excitotoxicity. A family of sodium-dependent Glu transporters particularly enriched in glial cells is responsible for the removal of this transmitter from the synaptic cleft [12]. These transporters, known as excitatory amino acid transporters (EAAT), are differentially expressed in neurons and astrocytes. EAAT3, 4, and 5 are mainly neuronal, whereas EAAT1 and EAAT2 are glial, although the latter one has also been found to be present in certain neuronal populations [18]. Once Glu has been taken up by glial cells, it is mostly converted to glutamine (Gln) by the glial-expressed Gln synthetase to be released in the vicinity of the presynaptic terminal, a process known as the Glu/Gln shuttle, in which an exquisite interplay between neurons and glial cells is fundamental for the proper function of glutamatergic transmission [12]. In this context, glutamatergic synapses are a perfect example of what has been lately known as a tripartite synapse [19].

3. Notch signaling

Notch signaling involves cell to cell communication and has a simple core. It initiates when the Notch receptor (Notch 1-4), present in the receiving-signal cell, binds its ligand (Jagged/Delta-like) present in the sending-signal cell. This binding promotes two sequential proteolytic cleavages on the Notch receptor: the first is mediated by the protease ADAM10/TACE (tumor necrosis factor α converting enzyme) to generate the membrane-tethered intermediated Notch extracellular truncation (NEXT). The second cleavage is mediated by the γ-Secretase enzyme on NEXT, to release the signal effector Notch intracellular domain (NICD) into the cytoplasm. NICD is translocated to the nucleus where it binds the transcription factor CSL (CBF1/RBPJκ in vertebrates, suppressor of hairless in *Drosophila*, Lag-1 in *C. elegans*) to activate what is known as the canonical Notch pathway. In the absence of NICD, CSL associates with the ubiquitous co-repressors (Co-R): SKIP, CtBP/Hairless, SMRT, CIR, FLH1C/KyoT2, SHARP/MINT and Gro/TLE proteins, and histone deacetylases (HDACs) to halt the transcription of Notch target genes. Once NICD binds CSL, allosteric changes may occur on CSL that facilitates displacement of transcriptional repressors. The transcriptional co-activator Mastermind (MAM) then recognizes the NICD/CSL interface, and this tri-protein complex recruits additional co-activators (Co-A) to promote transcription of target genes, as the astroglial markers shown in **Table 1** [20–27].

The noncanonical Notch signaling pathway is CSL-independent and can as well be either ligand-dependent or independent. Nevertheless, one has to keep in mind that the NICD/CSL complex is the major effector of Notch signaling. Several pieces of evidence have demonstrated that the Notch pathway may signal independently of CSL. It was first reported that Notch could signal via the RING-domain of E3 ubiquitin ligase Deltex1 (DTX1) [28]. It has also been shown that NEXT binds NICD on its ankyrin repeats [29], leading to its nuclear translocation. It has been documented as well that the NICD/DTX1 complex interacts with the transcriptional co-activator p300 inhibiting the transcriptional activation of the neural-specific transcription factor MASH1 [30]. As it will be described later, other genes important for astroglial differentiation are also targets of NICD/DTX (**Table 1**).

	Target	Function	Reference
Canonical pathway (NICD/ RBPJκ-dependent)	Hes1/Hes5	Down-regulate pro-neural transcription factors, as Mash1, Math, and Neurogenin; which in turns regulate neural protein expression (p. ej.MAP2)	[72]
	Glutamate aspartate transporter (GLAST)	Glutamate transport	This work
	(Glial fibrillary acidic protein (GFAP)	Principal protein (most abundant) forming an intermediate filament in mature astrocytes. Is important in radial glia cytoskeleton.	[50]
	Binding lipid-binding protein (BLBP)	Hydrophobic protein member from the family FABP (Fatty acid–binding protein). Binds to ligands of nuclear receptors and participate regulating their transcriptional activity.	[32, 33]
	Vimentin	Most abundant protein forming intermediate filaments in immature astrocytes and radial glia	[73]
Noncanonical (NICD/ RBPJκ-independent)	erbB2	Tyrosine kinase receptor	[33]
	Slug	Zinc-finger transcription factor that regulates neural crest formation and delamination	[74]
	β-catenin/Wnt signaling	Wnt/β-catenin signaling; Notch binds and titrates levels of the obligate Wnt-signaling component active β-catenin.	[75, 76]
	BMP4	Induce neural crest cells from the neural plate. Bmp4 can induce Slug expression and subsequent neural crest	[74, 77]

Table 1. Targets of Notch signaling pathway in central nervous system development.

4. Notch pathway signaling in astroglial differentiation

Notch pathway is a pivotal signaling system during neuro- and gliogenesis in the central nervous system (CNS) [24, 25]. Primary neural stem cells (NSC) are radial glia (RG) during development, characterized by the expression of astroglial markers such as the astrocyte-specific glutamate/aspartate transporter (GLAST), the brain lipid-binding protein (BLBP), and tenascin C (TN-C) [31]. RG cells generate neurons, oligodendrocytes, and astrocytes in a characteristic spatial and temporal pattern [31]. In this context, the Notch pathway plays an essential role repressing neurogenesis and maintaining the self-renewal potential of RG.

On the neurogenic phase, RG divide asymmetrically for auto-renewal and generation of neurons or neuron-restricted intermediate progenitor cells (nIPCs, transit amplifying cells), which in turn populate the subventricular zone (SVZ) in the cortex. The newborn neurons migrate along parental RG fibers, even though RG are dividing [31]. The Notch pathway plays an important role during the neurogenic phase in several ways. In the cortex, recent findings suggest that Notch signaling among SVZ nIPCs and between nIPCs and RG is important in the regulation of progenitor proliferation and in the inhibition of precocious neuronal differentiation. RG receives Notch signaling to activate Hes1 and Hes5 transcription factors, which down-regulate pro-neuronal genes such as neurogenin 1 (Ngn1), Mash1, and Math.

At the same time, Ngn1 becomes an astrogenesis inhibitor through the sequestration of p300/CBP, a key inducer of astrocyte differentiation [29].

In the cerebellum and in the immature RG, it has been demonstrated that Notch1 is activated by Jagged1 on newborn neuron progenitors; this interaction regulates the molecular and morphological differentiation of RG, through the transcriptional activation of BLBP and the erbB2 receptor tyrosine kinase. This effect is mediated by two downstream mechanisms, one that depends on RBPJκ (canonical activation) and the other depending on Deltex1 (DTX1) (noncanonical activation). In this manner, the induced erbB2 receptor interacts with its ligand neuregulin, present on neuronal progenitors, to facilitate cell migration through RG fibers (**Figure 1**) [32, 33].

After the neurogenesis period, at the end of embryonic development, most of the RG cells have lost their ventricular attachment and migrate toward the cortical plate by a process of somal translocation. In mammals, the majority of RG cells are transformed into astrocytes. During this period, astrocytic and oligodendrocytic intermediate precursors are also generated (aIPCs and oIPCs). Some studies suggest the presence of multipotent and bipotent progenitors, and perhaps astrocyte-restricted progenitors in the neonatal SVZ [34].

Astrogenesis depends on several stimuli, being the Notch pathway a master regulator of the differentiation process. During the gliogenic phase, RG progenitors gain competence to generate astrocytes due to the activity of growth factors such as basic fibroblast growth factor (bFGF) and epidermal growth factor (EGF). This gain of competence allows them to respond to specific gliogenic signals acting at the extracellular level to activate astrocyte markers such as glial fibrillary acidic protein (GFAP), S100β, aquaporin 4, glutamate transporters (GLT-1, EACC1, and GLAST), and aldehyde dehydrogenase 1 family, member L1 (AldhL1) [35–39]. Before the astrocyte-marker promoters can respond to gliogenic signals, a chromatin epigenetic remodeling must occur. Notch canonical activation on RG induces expression of nuclear factor 1A (NFA1), an inhibitor of the DNA methyltransferase 1 (DNMT1). DNMT1 keeps STAT3 site of GFAP promoter methylated and inactive [40, 41].

The extracellular signals are provided by neurotrophic cytokines such as ciliary neurotrophic factor (CNTF), leukemia inhibitory factor (LIF), and cardiotrophin-1 (CT-1) secreted by newborn neurons. These cytokines activate heterodimeric cell surface receptors composed of two subunits named LIFRβ and gp130, which in turn activate to members of the JAK family of tyrosine kinases that result in the phosphorylation and nuclear translocation of signal transducer and activator of transcription (STAT) proteins. In RG, two of these proteins, STAT1 and STAT3, act on specific sites in the promoters of the astroglial genes GFAP and S100β to stimulate their transcription during the astrocyte differentiation process. Neural progenitors also respond to different neurotrophic factors from the bone morphogenetic proteins (BMP) family to generate astrocytes. In this case, BMP2 and BMP4 act on heterotrimeric receptors, which activate SMAD transcription factors. These, in turn, interact with activated STAT proteins to synergistically stimulate transcription of glial-specific genes during astrocyte differentiation [42–47].

Another estrogen signal is the activation of the seven transmembrane domain G protein-coupled receptors by the pituitary adenylate cyclase-activating polypeptide (PACAP), triggering the differentiation of astrocytes by increasing intracellular cAMP and activating the cAMP-dependent protein kinase (PKA), which translocates into the nucleus to phosphorylate and

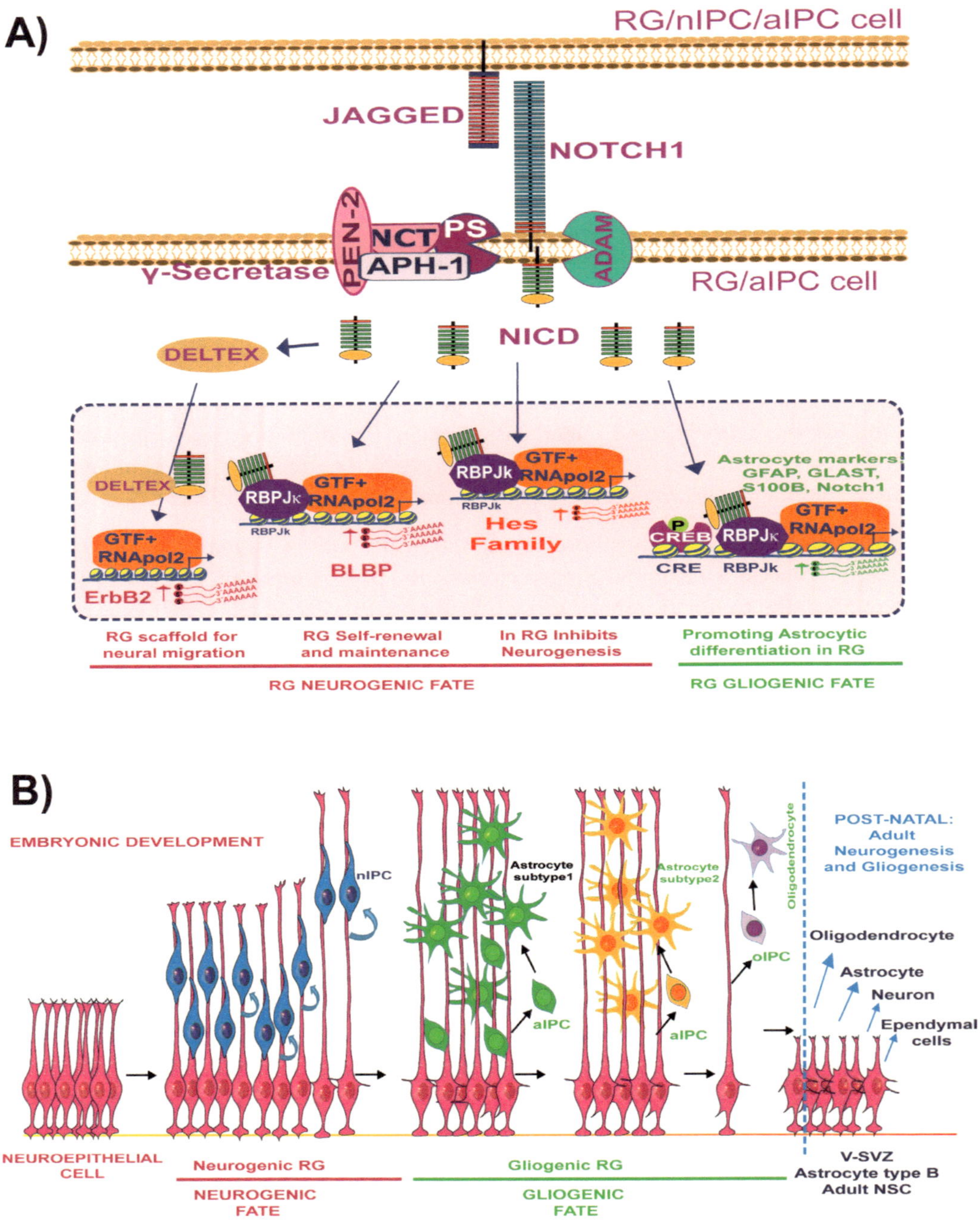

Figure 1. Notch pathway regulates astrocytic differentiation. (A) In timed cell genesis, a series of orchestrated events are activated to regulate cell differentiation; the Notch pathway is used as a signaling system during embryonic development and regulates different cell markers in astrocyte differentiation, such as Hes genes, GFAP and S100B. (nIPC/aIPC cell stands for neural or astrocytic intermediate precursor cell). (B) Neuroepithelial cells in early development proliferate by asymmetric cell division to generate more neuroepithelial cells (progenitor expansion phase). As brain development proceeds, neuroepithelial cells elongate to convert into radial glial (RG) cells and guide neuronal migration. Later, RG can divide asymmetrically to generate neuron, astrocyte, or oligodendrocyte intermediate progenitor cells.

activate the cAMP-response element-binding protein (CREB) [42–48]. In a glial precursor-like model, C6 cells, cAMP-PKA-CREB activation leads to increase autocrine IL-6, which in turn activates STAT3, which induces GFAP promoter activation [49]. In the same model, the cAMP-PKA-CREB signaling cascade cross talks with the Notch pathway, and together they act synergistically to reduce the progenitor marker (Nestin) and to induce astrocytic differentiation; measured by induced astrocytic markers (GFAP, S100β, and GLAST) and glutamate uptake. In this context, Notch1 mRNA is up-regulated in a PKA/γ-secretase/NICD/CSL-dependent manner, suggesting the establishment of a feedback loop to keep Notch pathway active until astrocytic differentiation is complete [50]. It is not surprising that the Notch pathway interacts with other signaling cascades to complete astrocytic differentiation. A bioinformatic analysis of promoters for GFAP, S100β, GLAST, and Notch1, reveals specific sites for CREB, STAT3, and CSL transcription factors, suggesting that these three pathways, cAMP-PKA/JAK-STAT3/Notch, cooperate to induce the transcription of astrocyte markers. Certainly, at this stage, other crosstalk interactions cannot be discarded.

5. Glial differentiation and the Ca^{2+}/diacylglycerol-dependent protein kinase (PKC)

As already mentioned, glial differentiation is modulated by extracellular signals, growth factors, hormones, cytokines, neurotrophins, and neurotransmitters that activate different signal pathways. PKC is one of the major mediators of these extracellular signals. The structure of this family of protein kinases contains a highly conserved catalytic domain and a regulatory domain (C1-C4 domains) responsible for its inactive conformation. Regulatory domains are separated by variable regions susceptible to proteolytic cleavage and essential for activation and conformational changes. The PKC family comprises 11 isoforms and is organized in three subfamilies: classical, novel, and atypical isoforms described in **Table 2** [51–54].

PKC is highly expressed in the brain, with a significant role of this kinase in the function of neuronal and glial cells. The role of PKC in glial cells has been demonstrated in different reports, and PKC-activator PMA as well as the different PKC inhibitors, modify the cell morphology, proliferation, and differentiation [55–58]. Differential expression of PKC isoforms has been reported during neuronal development as four PKC isoforms are expressed in neuronal primary cultures of rat cerebellum. In contrast, only two isoforms, αPKC and βII PKC, are present in glial cultures [59, 60]. Brodie et al. reported that in undifferentiated C6 cells, the PKC isoforms θ, μ, ζ, and λ are present; however, the cAMP-dependent differentiated C6 cells expressed significantly lower levels of PKC α and PKC δ and higher levels of PKC γ, η, and θ.

Concerning PKC and glial cell function, overexpression of the β and γ isoforms increases GFAP levels, as a response to exposure to the PKC activator phorbol 12-myristate 13-acetate (PMA) treatment. Glutamine synthetase (GS) levels increase with PKC γ overexpression and decrease with PKC δ. Therefore, it is plausible that PKC α and δ provide negative signals for astrocytic differentiation, while PKC β and γ induce astrocyte differentiation [51].

However, it has also been documented that undifferentiated C6 cells express the α, βII, γ, δ, ε, and ζ PKC isoforms and that long-term PKC inhibition after staurosporine treatment, which

	Isoforms	Activity
Classical isoforms	α, βI, βII, γ	Dependent on DAG, PS, and Ca^{2+}
Novel PKC isoforms	δ, ε, θ, η, μ	Bind DAG, PS, and calcium-independent
Atypical PKC isoforms	ι/λ, ξ	Bind PIP3, calcium-independent and do not require DAG
Diacylglycerol (DAG), phosphatidylserine (PS), phosphatidylinositol 3-phosphate (PIP3) [53, 78].		

Table 2. PKC classification.

leads to differentiation, results in βII decrease, γ increase and ε translocation from the membrane to the cytosol [55]. Similar results were reported in the C6 cell differentiation process with dbcAMP [61]. It is clear that the molecular mechanisms triggered by glia differentiation agents are different, but that the various PKC isoforms are critically involved in the overall process.

In contrast, Watanabe et al. recently reported that overexpression of PKC βII synergistically enhanced differentiation in the presence of 1 nM of PACAP. These results indicate that the β isoform of PKC is important in PACAP-induced differentiation of mouse embryonic NSCs into astrocytes via the PAC1 receptor, resulting in activation of phospholipase C, followed by PKC activation. This latter observation was confirmed in NSCs. The cells were exposed to 2 nM PACAP, resulting in a transient increase in the βII isoform, that returned to basal levels by day 4, whereas the levels of PKC α increased linearly up to day 6 [62].

RG cells and astrocytes are involved in regulation of the brain microenvironment, and glutamate transporters control the extracellular levels of this neurotransmitter. Regulation of glutamate uptake involves several factors like neuronal interactions, glutamate, cAMP, and phorbol esters. GLAST is the major glutamate transporter expressed in RG cells. Interestingly, GLAST expression is regulated via PKC through the reduction of its protein and mRNA levels. Our work group demonstrated that *chglast* transcriptional regulation is mediated by PKC, especially the α and ε isoforms, which activate the AP-1 transcription factor [56, 63, 64].

6. Another Notch in the belt: PKC/Notch cross talk in glial differentiation

The Notch signaling pathway plays an important role in the control of cell fate during developmental processes. Several reports have shown that Notch-induced signaling interacts with other signaling pathways, such as NF-κB, the mitogen-activated protein kinase (MAPK) pathway, and the phosphatidylinositol 3-kinase (PI3K)/Akt pathway [65–67]. Although there are only a few reports describing the crosstalk between Notch and PKC signaling during glial differentiation, some connections have been described so far. The most direct example concerns the direct PKC action over NICD: Kim et al. found that PKC δ down-regulates NICD transcriptional activity in a kinase-independent manner. The mechanism involves the inhibition of the nuclear localization of NICD, most possibly through a physical association between NICD and PKCδ causing the dissociation of NICD from target gene promoters like Hes5 [67].

In another example, PMA increased the expression of Notch1 in a PKCε-dependent manner in the context of astrocytic differentiation, and this is to say that in the course of PKC-dependent astrocyte differentiation, an increase in Notch levels is found. In fact, serine 729 PKCε phosphorylation is as essential for the differentiation process. This data suggests that Notch1 is a plausible mediator of PKCε in astrocytic differentiation [68]. In the same line, Xu et al. reported that morphine-dependent astrocytic differentiation of neuronal progenitor cells (NPC) involves ERK via PKCε and TRBP phosphorylation that leads to miR-181a maturation, thus regulating the expression of Prox1 and Notch1 [69].

More recently, it has been demonstrated that atypical PKC isoforms participate in asymmetric cell division when glial differentiation starts. Sjoqvist et al. demonstrated that PKCζ regulates the Notch pathway by phosphorylation and regulation of Notch receptor traffic. When Notch signaling is active (after ligand stimulation or after expression of an activated membrane-tethered form of Notch), PKCζ enhances the production of NICD and shifts the localization of Notch from late endosomes to the nucleus, leading to an elevated Notch signaling. In contrast, when the Notch receptor is not activated, PKCζ interacts with the receptor to induce a shift in receptor distribution from the plasma membrane to intracellular vesicles [70]. In C6 glioma cells, increased cAMP levels promote astrocytic commitment with a sustained augmentation of Notch activity, as detected by nuclear translocation of its intracellular domain portion (NICD) and its transcriptional activity [50]. The cAMP effect is mediated through the activation of the γ-secretase complex, responsible for Notch cleavage as demonstrated by its sensitivity to PKA inhibitors. As expected, Notch cleavage and nuclear translocation result in the upregulation of the mRNA levels of one of its target genes, the transcription factor Hair, and enhancer of split 5. Moreover, glutamate uptake activity, expression of astrocytic markers (genes responsible for glial progenitor cell fate decision) such as the glial fibrillary acidic protein, the S100beta protein, and GLAST, are also enhanced in cAMP-exposed cells [50]. Interestingly, polychlorinated biphenyls (PCBs) disturb the cAMP-induced astrocytic differentiation of C6 cells via the PKC isoforms γ, β2, δ and ε [58]. Additionally, PMA promotes adult neurogenesis by inducing neural progenitor cell proliferation *in vitro* in NPCs obtained from the SVZ of 7-day postnatal mice [71].

To support a plausible role of a crosstalk between PKC and Notch pathways in embryonic glial differentiation, we used chick Bergman radial glia from cerebellum (BGC) at day 14 of embryonic development and stimulated PKC using TPA. In this system, it was observed that PKC activation increased NICD/RPBJκ-dependent transcription, measured by a reporter construct that senses directly the CSL activity (**Figure 2A**). This effect could be mediated by the classical PKC isoforms (α, β1, β2, and γ) and/or the novel isoforms (δ and ε), as it was observed when the specific inhibitor bisindolylmaleimide 1 (Bis1). The same effect was observed over a Hes1-responsive reporter (**Figure 2A**, right). Also, the MAPK/ERK pathway plays a role in PKC-mediated NICD/RPBJκ activation, as demonstrated when specific MAPK/ERK inhibitors (U0126, PD98059, and SB202190) were used in co-treatment with TPA (**Figure 2A**). In contrast, treatment of BGC with TPA, down-regulates astrocytic biomarkers such as GFAP, GS, GLAST, FABP7, and Notch1 mRNA levels, and keeps Nestin, a progenitor marker, up-regulated (**Figure 2B**). Our results suggest that the activation of PKC induces NICD/RBPJκ dependent transcriptional activation by a yet-to-be characterized mechanism, that perhaps

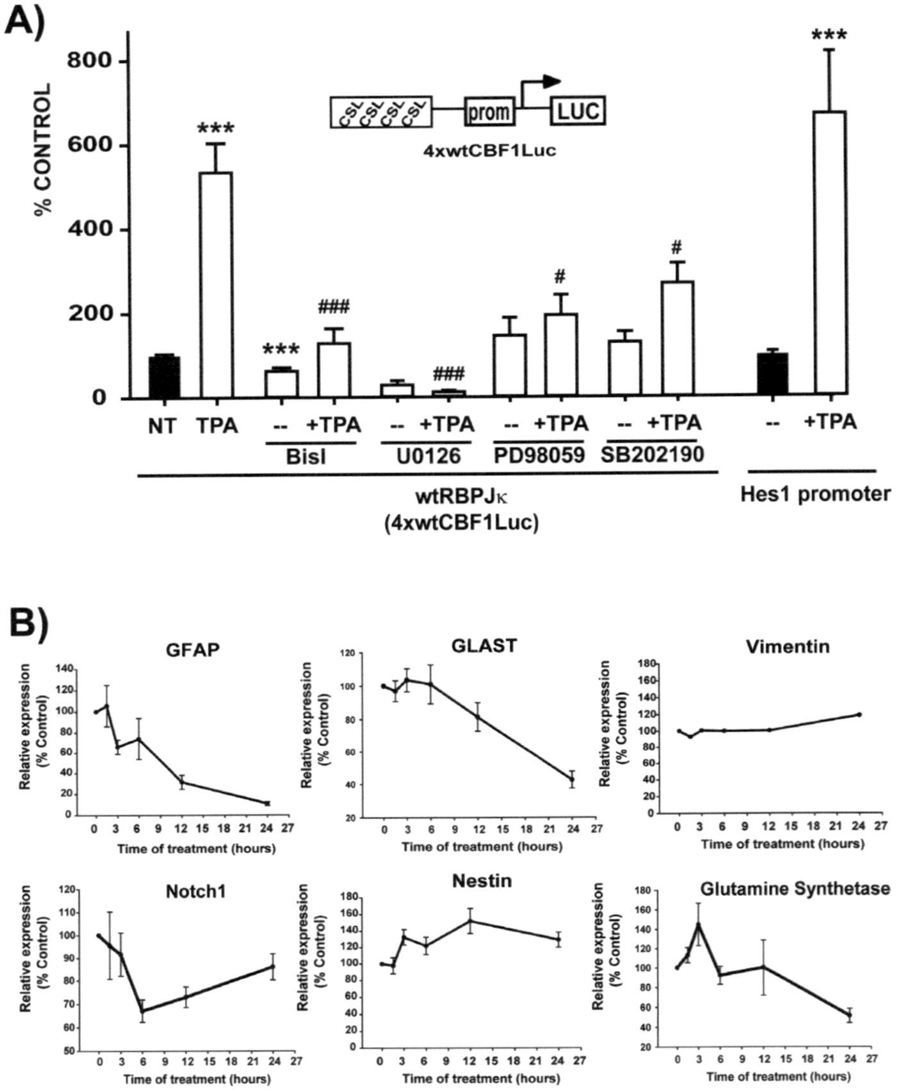

Figure 2. PKC/MAPK signaling activates Notch pathway in cultured Bergmann glia cells (BGCs). (A) In order to determine the role of the Notch/PKC signaling pathway in BGCs, cells (primary culture) were transfected with the reporter plasmid 4xwtCBF1Luc (containing four repeated sequences for RBPJκ elements) or Hes1 promoter (a Notch effector gene) with Lipofectamine R 2000; after harvesting, the luciferase reporter activity was measured. 24 h post-transfection, the BGCs were treated with 100 nM TPA for other 24 h, where we showed that promoter activity increased five-fold in relation with nontreatment cells, and TPA induces the Notch signaling response. To analyze the signal pathway involved in Notch activation, BGCs were treated with 40 μM BisI (a PKC inhibitor), 50 μM U0126 (a MAPK1 inhibitor), PD (PD8059, a MAPK1 inhibitor), or SB20 (SB202190, a specific ERK inhibitor) 30 min prior to TPA, as indicated in the figure. Note that both PKC and MAPK inhibitors prevent Notch pathway activation. Results are presented as fold expression relative to nontreated cells. Data represent mean values ± SE (n = 3). Data were analyzed by a one-way ANOVA with a post hoc Dunn's test. *** $p < 0.001$; ### $p < 0.003$; #, $p < 0.05$. (B) qRT-PCR was performed to analyze expression of Notch pathway targets, and BGC cultures were treated or not with TPA (100 nM TPA) at different times. Total RNA was extracted to amplify GFAP, GLAST, vimentin, glutamine synthetase (astrocytic markers), and nestin (radial glial marker) with the KAPA SYBR FAST one-step qRT-PCR kit. Our data suggest that TPA downregulates GLAST, GFAP, and GS and upregulates nestin; this evidence indicates that the Notch pathway is important in the radial glial fate.

http://dx.doi.org/10.5772/intechopen.73318

is related to regulation of NICD routing and trafficking [67, 70]. The NICD/RBPJκ complex induces Hes1 expression, a well-known neurogenesis inhibitor. On the other hand, PKC activation blocks astrogenesis, perhaps modulating the access of NICD/RBPJκ to the astrocytic markers' promoters, like GFAP, which is dependent on Notch activation. In BGC, PKC activation regulates several genes that are closely related to glial function and induces radial glial phenotype as TPA down-regulates GLAST, GFAP, and GS and upregulates Nestin, PKCα, or PKCε (PKC ◎2).

6.1. Notch pathway in CNS: some aspects of clinical relevance

A plethora of pathological scenarios in the CNS are the result of neuronal degeneration. This cell loss needs to be compensated to keep the neural circuits working. In this context, neural stem cells can be differentiated into precise neuronal subtypes, but a common fact is that Notch signaling promotes astrocyte differentiation rather than neuronal differentiation. Therefore, Notch inhibition is an alternative therapeutic option in the clinical approach. Examples of the possible application of inhibiting Notch are presented in the **Table 3**.

Pathological context/ biological system	**Targeted neural stem cells**	**Notch signaling role and possible therapeutic approach**	**Ref**
Blockage of notch pathway in neural adult stem cells to promote neurogenesis			
Glioblastoma (multiforme or grade IV astrocytoma)	Glioblastoma cells (GB)	Pharmacological inhibition of Notch pathway selectively inhibited tumor growth. Conversely, activation of Notch signaling promotes cell proliferation and colony formation in the human GB cell line. Notch1 promotes invasive migratory properties of GB cells by stimulating β-catenin and NF-κB signaling and mediates GB cell proliferation and survival through the Akt-mammalian target of rapamycin (mTOR) signaling axis. Treatment with γ-secretase inhibitors reduces neurosphere growth, and inhibits xenograft tumor growth through decreased Akt and STAT3 phosphorylation. Combination of Notch inhibitor MRK003 and Akt inhibitor MK-2206 effectively inhibited GB invasiveness.	[79]
Lineage-specific differentiation of NPCs	Hippocampal progenitor cells (HPC)	Phosphorylation of TAR RNA-binding protein together with miR-181a maturation, as well as Dicer activity, is involved in morphine-induced astrocyte-preferential differentiation of HPC.	[69]
Alzheimer's disease (AD) Amyloid precursor protein (APP)	Human neural progenitor cells (HNPC)	Activation of IL-6/gp130 and Notch signaling pathways in glial differentiation of HNPCs may cause problems in maintaining normal brain function and may contribute to AD pathology. Treatment with sAPP increased expression levels of GFAP in NT-2/D1 cells along with the generation of Notch intracellular domain (NICD) and expression of Hairy and enhancer of split 1 (Hes1), indicating that glial differentiation may aid in the development of novel therapeutic strategies for AD.	[80] [81]
Blood-brain barrier, pathology	Brain endothelial cells	Neuron-derived Dll1 activates Notch signaling and is essential for brain endothelial cells' survival as wells as blood-brain barrier, selective substance crossing; physiology, pathology, and drug development	[82]

Pathological context/ biological system	Targeted neural stem cells	Notch signaling role and possible therapeutic approach	Ref
Traumatic brain injury (TBI), inflammation and apoptosis and brain edema	Cerebral cortices response	Inhibition of Notch signaling by crocin, an extract of saffron, has a neuroprotective effect against TBI, since in this type of injury an upregulation of Notch intracellular domain (NICD) and Hes1 mRNA levels is present, decreasing microglial activation and release of several pro-inflammatory cytokines.	[83]
Increased differentiation of neural progenitor cells when co-cultured with astrocytes lacking glial fibrillary acidic protein (GFAP) and vimentin	Neural progenitor cells	Astrocytes negatively regulate neurogenesis through Notch pathway; endocytosis of Notch ligand Jagged1 in astrocytes and Notch signaling from astrocytes to neural stem/progenitor cells depends on intermediate filament proteins GFAP and vimentin.	[84]
Experimental autoimmune encephalomyelitis (failure to repair demyelination) as Multiple Sclerosis model (mice)	Oligodendrocyte precursor cells	Gamma-secretase inhibition of Notch signaling enhances tissue repair. Notch pathway inhibits oligodendrocytes differentiation and hampers their ability to produce myelin during CNS development.	[85, 86]
Seizure as a serious complication of stroke	Neurons in cortex and hippo-campus	In a global cerebral ischemia model (GCI), there is augmented excitatory synaptic neurotransmission by upregulating glutamate receptor subunits (GluN2A, GluA1) and cotransporter NKCC1, but there is attenuated inhibitory synaptic neurotransmission by down-regulating amino butyric acid (GABA), and neuronal K-Cl cotransporter. Aberrant activation of Notch signaling is involved in poststroke seizures, as NICD 1 and 2 were upregulated in the cerebral cortex and hippocampus post-GCI. DAPT treatment normalized the homeostasis of excitatory and inhibitory synaptic neurotransmission.	[87]
Familial and idiopathic Parkinson's disease (PD)	Differentiated dopaminergic neurons	Leucine-rich repeat kinase 2 (LRRK2) complex promotes recycling of Notch ligand Delta-like 1 (Dll1)/Delta (Dl) through modulation of endosomal trafficking and negatively regulates Notch signaling through *cis*-inhibition by stabilizing Dll1/Dl, accelerating neural stem cell differentiation; alteration of Notch signaling in mature neurons is a component of PD etiology linked to *LRRK2*.	[88]
Notch signaling in neurodegenerative diseases and pathological glutamate mediated plasticity			
Dopamine release in the striatum, individual's susceptibility to neuropsychiatric disease	Neuronal cells	RBP-J deficiency drastically reduced dopamine release in the striatum and caused a subtle decrease in the number of dopaminergic neurons as Notch/RBP-J signaling regulates dopamine responsiveness in the striatum.	[89].
Length, polarity, and synaptogenesis	Spiral ganglion neurons (SGNs)	DNER modulates length, polarity and synaptogenesis *via* the Notch signaling pathway. DNER was expressed in spiral ganglion neurons exhibiting significant polarity in early differentiation stages; DNER expression gradually decreased until polarity was lost on week 35. Silencing DNER expression altered the polarity of differentiated neurons and these cells exhibited significantly reduced dendritic length.	[90]

Table 3. Notch signaling in cell therapy.

7. Conclusion

Glia cells play an active role in glutamatergic transmission due to their compulsory intervention in the recycling of this excitatory neurotransmitter. The Notch signal transduction pathway is critically involved in the gene expression regulation of the major excitatory amino acid transporter expressed in early stages of astrocyte differentiation and in RG in the adult brain. Notch signaling involves the activation of diverse isoforms of PKC. Glial differentiation can be mediated by PKC and its isoforms, which act over NICD, increasing Notch expression, regulating several astrocytic markers related to glial function, and inducing the radial glial phenotype.

Acknowledgements

The work in our labs is funded by Conacyt-Mexico 255087 and Soluciones para un México Verde, S.A. de C.V. granted to AO and Conacyt-PEI 212650 and 231793 granted to ELB.

Conflict of interest

The authors declare that there are no conflicts of interest.

Abbreviations

ADAM10/TACE	Tumor necrosis factor-α converting enzyme
AldhL1	aldehyde dehydrogenase 1
bFGF	Basic fibroblast growth factor
BGC	Chick Bergmann Radial glia
BisI	Bisindolylmaleimide
BLBP	Brain lipid-binding protein
BMP	Bone morphogenetic proteins
cAMP	Cyclic adenosine monophosphate
CIR	Corepressor interacting with RBPJ 1
CNS	Central nervous system
CNTF	Ciliary neurotrophic factor

CREB	cAMP-response element-binding protein
CT-1	Cardiotrophin-1
DNMT1	DNA methyl transferase 1
DTX1	Deltex1
EAATs	Excitatory amino acid transporters
EACC1	Excitatory amino acid transporter 1
EGF	Epidermal growth factor
ErbB2	also known as HER2, Human epidermal growth factor receptor 2
ERK	Extracellular signal-regulated kinases
FABP7	Fatty acid–binding protein 7
GFAP	Glial fibrillary acidic protein
GLAST	Glutamate aspartate transporter
GLT-1	Glutamate transporter 1
GS	Glutamine synthetase
HDAC	Histone deacetylases
LIF	Leukemia inhibitory factor
LIFRβ	Leukemia inhibitory factor receptor β
MAM	Mastermind
MAP 2	Microtubule-associated protein 2
MAPK	Mitogen-activated protein kinase
MASH	Mammalian achaete-scute homolog-1
NEXT	Notch extracellular truncation
NFA1	Nuclear factor 1A
NF-κB	Nuclear factor kappa-light-chain-enhancer of activated B cells
Ngn1	Neurogenin 1
NICD	Notch intracellular domain
NIPC	Intermediate progenitor cell

PACAP	Pituitary adenylate cyclase-activating polypeptide
PI3K	Phosphatidylinositol 3-kinase
PKA	cAMP-dependent protein kinase
PKC	Protein kinase C
PMA	Phorbol 12-myristate 13-acetate
RBPJκ	Recombining binding protein
RG	Radial glia
SMRT	Thyroid-hormone receptors
STAT3	Signal transducer and activator of transcription 3
SVZ	Subventricular Zone
TN-C	Tenascin C
TPA	12-O-tetradecanoylphorbol 13-acetate
TRBP	TAR RNA-binding protein

Author details

López-Bayghen Esther[1], Angulo-Rojo Carla[2], López-Bayghen Bruno[1], Hernández-Melchor Dinorah[1], Ramírez Leticia[1] and Ortega Arturo[1*]

*Address all correspondence to: arortega@cinvestav.mx

1 Departamento de Toxicología, Centro de Investigación de Estudios Avanzados del IPN, México City, Mexico

2 Unidad de Investigación, Facultad de Medicina, Universidad Autónoma de Sinaloa, Culiacán, Sinaloa, Mexico

References

[1] Gasic GP et al. Molecular neurobiology of glutamate receptors. Annual Review of Physiology. 1992;**54**:507-536. DOI: 10.1146/annurev.ph.54.030192.002451

[2] Hollmann M et al. Cloned glutamate receptors. Annual Review of Neuroscience. 1994;**17**: 31-108. DOI: 10.1146/annurev.ne.17.030194.000335

[3] Schoepp DD et al. Metabotropic glutamate receptors and neuronal degenerative disorders. Neurobiology of Aging. 1994;**15**(2):261-263

[4] Pin JP et al. The metabotropic glutamate receptors: Structure and functions. Neuropharmacology. 1995;**34**(1):1-26

[5] Cameron RS et al. Glial cell lineage in the cerebral cortex: A review and synthesis. Glia. 1991;**4**(2):124-137. DOI: 10.1002/glia.440040204

[6] Malatesta P et al. Neuronal or glial progeny: Regional differences in radial glia fate. Neuron. 2003;**37**(5):751-764

[7] Anthony TE et al. Radial glia serve as neuronal progenitors in all regions of the central nervous system. Neuron. 2004;**41**(6):881-890

[8] Danbolt NC. Glutamate uptake. Progress in Neurobiology. 2001;**65**(1):1-105

[9] Eulenburg V et al. Neurotransmitter transporters expressed in glial cells as regulators of synapse function. Brain Research Reviews. 2010;**63**(1-2):103-112. DOI: 10.1016/j.brainresrev.2010.01.003

[10] Swanson CJ et al. Metabotropic glutamate receptors as novel targets for anxiety and stress disorders. Nature Reviews. Drug Discovery. 2005;**4**(2):131-144. DOI: 10.1038/nrd1630

[11] Maragakis NJ et al. Glutamate transporter expression and function in human glial progenitors. Glia. 2004;**45**(2):133-143. DOI: 10.1002/glia.10310

[12] Martinez-Lozada Z et al. Glutamatergic transmission: A matter of three. Neural Plasticity. 2015;**2015**:787396. DOI: 10.1155/2015/787396

[13] Araque A et al. Glial modulation of synaptic transmission in culture. Glia. 2004;**47**(3):241-248. DOI: 10.1002/glia.20026

[14] Gonzalez MI et al. Regulation of high-affinity glutamate uptake activity in Bergmann glia cells by glutamate. Brain Research. 2000;**866**(1-2):73-81

[15] Gegelashvili M et al. Glutamate transporter Glast/Eaat1 directs cell surface expression of Fxyd2/gamma subunit of Na, K-Atpase in human fetal astrocytes. Neurochemistry International. 2007;**50**(7-8):916-920. DOI: 10.1016/j.neuint.2006.12.015

[16] Rose EM et al. Glutamate transporter coupling to Na,K-Atpase. The Journal of Neuroscience. 2009;**29**(25):8143-8155. DOI: 10.1523/JNEUROSCI.1081-09.2009

[17] Martinez-Lozada Z et al. Glast/Eaat1-induced glutamine release via Snat3 in Bergmann glial cells: Evidence of a functional and physical coupling. Journal of Neurochemistry. 2013;**125**(4):545-554. DOI: 10.1111/jnc.12211

[18] Danbolt NC et al. Neuronal vs glial glutamate uptake: Resolving the conundrum. Neurochemistry International. 2016;**98**:29-45. DOI: 10.1016/j.neuint.2016.05.009

[19] Flores-Mendez M et al. Glia plasma membrane transporters: Key players in Glutamatergic neurotransmission. Neurochemistry International. 2016;**98**:46-55. DOI: 10.1016/j.neuint.2016.04.004

[20] Fortini ME. Notch and presenilin: A proteolytic mechanism emerges. Current Opinion in Cell Biology. 2001;**13**(5):627-634. DOI: 10.1016/S0955-0674(00)00261-1

[21] Fortini ME. Gamma-secretase-mediated proteolysis in cell-surface-receptor signalling. Nature Reviews. Molecular Cell Biology. 2002;**3**(9):673-684. DOI: 10.1038/nrm910

[22] Fortini ME et al. The suppressor of hairless protein participates in notch receptor signaling. Cell. 1994;**79**(2):273-282. DOI: 10.1016/0092-8674(94)90196-1

[23] Kopan R et al. The canonical notch signaling pathway: Unfolding the activation mechanism. Cell. 2009;**137**(2):216-233. DOI: 10.1016/j.cell.2009.03.045

[24] Bray SJ. Notch signalling: A simple pathway becomes complex. Nature Reviews. Molecular Cell Biology. 2006;**7**(9):678-689. DOI: 10.1038/nrm2009

[25] Chiba S. Concise review: Notch signaling in stem cell systems. Stem Cells. 2006;**24**(11): 2437-2447. DOI: 10.1634/stemcells.2005-0661

[26] Selkoe D et al. Notch and presenilin: Regulated intramembrane proteolysis links development and degeneration. Annual Review of Neuroscience. 2003;**26**(1):565-597. DOI: 10.1146/annurev.neuro.26.041002.131334

[27] Mumm JS et al. Notch signaling: From the outside in. Developmental Biology. 2000; **228**(2):151-165. DOI: 10.1006/dbio.2000.9960

[28] Gorman MJ et al. A genetic analysis of Deltex and its interaction with the notch locus in drosophila melanogaster. Genetics. 1992;**131**(1):99-112

[29] Matsuno K et al. Deltex acts as a positive regulator of notch signaling through interactions with the notch Ankyrin repeats. Development. 1995;**121**(8):2633-2644

[30] Yamamoto N et al. Role of Deltex-1 as a transcriptional regulator downstream of the notch receptor. The Journal of Biological Chemistry. 2001;**276**(48):45031-45040. DOI: 10.1074/jbc.M105245200

[31] Kriegstein A et al. The glial nature of embryonic and adult neural stem cells. Annual Review of Neuroscience. 2009;**32**:149-184. DOI: 10.1146/annurev.neuro.051508.135600

[32] Patten BA et al. Sequential signaling through Notch1 and Erbb receptors mediates radial glia differentiation. The Journal of Neuroscience. 2003;**23**(14):6132-6140 23/14/6132 [pii]

[33] Patten BA et al. Notch1 signaling regulates radial glia differentiation through multiple transcriptional mechanisms. The Journal of Neuroscience. 2006;**26**(12):3102-3108. DOI: 10.1523/JNEUROSCI.4829-05.2006

[34] Aguirre A et al. Postnatal neurogenesis and gliogenesis in the olfactory bulb from Ng2-expressing progenitors of the subventricular zone. The Journal of Neuroscience. 2004;**24**(46):10530-10541. DOI: 10.1523/jneurosci.3572-04.2004

[35] Spassky N et al. Adult ependymal cells are postmitotic and are derived from radial glial cells during embryogenesis. The Journal of Neuroscience. 2005;**25**(1):10-18. DOI: 10.1523/jneurosci.1108-04.2005

[36] Wang DD et al. The astrocyte odyssey. Progress in Neurobiology. 2008;**86**(4):342-367. DOI: 10.1016/j.pneurobio.2008.09.015

[37] Liu X et al. Gfap-expressing cells in the postnatal subventricular zone display a unique glial phenotype intermediate between radial glia and astrocytes. Glia. 2006;**54**(5):394-410. DOI: 10.1002/glia.20392

[38] Kimelberg HK. The problem of astrocyte identity. Neurochemistry International. 2004; **45**(2-3):191-202. DOI: 10.1016/j.neuint.2003.08.015

[39] Cahoy JD et al. A transcriptome database for astrocytes, neurons, and oligodendrocytes: A new resource for understanding brain development and function. The Journal of Neuroscience. 2008;**28**(1):264-278. DOI: 10.1523/jneurosci.4178-07.2008

[40] Wilczynska KM et al. Nuclear factor I isoforms regulate gene expression during the differentiation of human neural progenitors to astrocytes. Stem Cells. 2009;**27**(5):1173-1181. DOI: 10.1002/stem.35

[41] Cebolla B et al. Nuclear factor-I regulates glial fibrillary acidic protein gene expression in astrocytes differentiated from cortical precursor cells. Journal of Neurochemistry. 2006;**97**(4):1057-1070. DOI: 10.1111/j.1471-4159.2006.03804.x

[42] Vallejo I et al. Pituitary adenylate cyclase-activating polypeptide induces astrocyte differentiation of precursor cells from developing cerebral cortex. Molecular and Cellular Neurosciences. 2002;**21**(4):671-683. DOI: 10.1006/mcne.2002.1189

[43] Jozwiak-Bebenista M et al. Effects of Pacap, Vip and related peptides on cyclic amp formation in rat neuronal and astrocyte cultures and cerebral cortical slices. Pharmacological Reports. 2007;**59**(4):414-420. DOI: 10.1016/j.peptides.2007.04.007

[44] Vallejo M. Pacap signaling to dream: A camp-dependent pathway that regulates cortical Astrogliogenesis. Molecular Neurobiology. 2009;**39**(2):90-100. DOI: 10.1007/s12035-009-8055-2

[45] Tatsuno I et al. Pituitary adenylate cyclase-activating polypeptide (Pacap) is a regulator of astrocytes: Pacap stimulates proliferation and production of interleukin 6 (Il-6), but not nerve growth factor (Ngf), in cultured rat astrocyte. Annals of the New York Academy of Sciences. 1996;**805**:482-488. DOI: 10.1111/j.1749-6632.1996.tb17508.x

[46] Nakamachi T et al. Role of Pacap in neural stem/progenitor cell and astrocyte: From neural development to neural repair. Current Pharmaceutical Design. 2011;**17**(10):973-984. DOI: 10.2174/138161211795589346

[47] Nakamachi T et al. Pituitary adenylate cyclase-activating polypeptide (Pacap) type 1 receptor (Pac1r) co-localizes with activity-dependent Neuroprotective protein (Adnp) in the mouse brains. Regulatory Peptides. 2008;**145**(1):88-95. DOI: 10.1016/j.regpep.2007.09.025

[48] Sands WA et al. Regulating gene transcription in response to cyclic amp elevation. Cellular Signalling. 2008;**20**(3):460-466. DOI: 10.1016/j.cellsig.2007.10.005

[49] Takanaga H et al. Camp-induced astrocytic differentiation of C6 Glioma cells is mediated by Autocrine Interleukin-6. The Journal of Biological Chemistry. 2004;**279**(15):15441-15447. DOI: 10.1074/jbc.M311844200

[50] Angulo-Rojo C et al. Involvement of the notch pathway in terminal astrocytic differentiation: Role of Pka. ASN Neuro. 2013;**5**(5):e00130. DOI: 10.1042/AN20130023

[51] Brodie C et al. Differential role of specific Pkc isoforms in the proliferation of glial cells and the expression of the astrocytic markers Gfap and glutamine Synthetase. Molecular Brain Research. 1998;**56**(1):108-117. DOI: 10.1016/S0169-328X(98)00035-7

[52] Nishizuka Y. Protein kinase C and lipid signaling for sustained cellular responses. The FASEB Journal. 1995;**9**(7):484-496

[53] Newton AC. Protein kinase C: Structure, function, and regulation. The Journal of Biological Chemistry. 1995;**270**(48):28495-28498. DOI: 10.1074/jbc.270.48.28495

[54] do Carmo A et al. Pkc signaling in glioblastoma. Cancer Biology & Therapy. 2013;**14**(4): 287-294. Doi: 10.4161/cbt.23615

[55] Kronfeld I et al. Staurosporine induces astrocytic phenotypes and differential expression of specific Pkc isoforms in C6 glial cells. Journal of Neurochemistry. 1995;**65**(4):1505-1514. DOI: 10.1046/j.1471-4159.1995.65041505.x

[56] Lopez-Bayghen E et al. Glutamate-dependent transcriptional regulation of Glast: Role of Pkc. Journal of Neurochemistry. 2004;**91**(1):200-209. DOI: 10.1111/j.1471-4159.2004.02706.x

[57] Moreton K et al. Protein expression of the A, Γ, Δ and E subspecies of protein kinase C changes as C6 Glioma cells become contact inhibited and quiescent in the presence of serum. FEBS Letters. 1995;**372**(1):33-38 https://doi.org/10.1016/0014-5793(95)00941-2

[58] Adornetto A et al. Polychlorinated biphenyls impair Dibutyryl camp-induced astrocytic differentiation in rat C6 glial cell line. FEBS Open Bio. 2013;**3**:459-466. DOI: 10.1016/j.fob.2013.10.008

[59] Masliah E et al. Differential involvement of protein kinase C Isozymes in Alzheimer's disease. The Journal of Neuroscience. 1990;**10**(7):2113-2124

[60] Moreton K et al. Changes in Pkc subspecies protein expression as C6 cells reach G(0) by contact inhibition in the presence of serum. Biochemical Society Transactions. 1995; **23**(3):446S)

[61] S-i Y et al. Differential expression of rho family Gtp-binding proteins and protein kinase C Isozymes during C6 glial cell differentiation. Molecular Brain Research. 1997;**45**(1): 90-98. DOI: 10.1016/S0169-328X(96)00239-2

[62] Watanabe J et al. Pituitary adenylate cyclase-activating polypeptide-induced differentiation of embryonic neural stem cells into astrocytes is mediated via the Beta isoform of

protein kinase C. Journal of Neuroscience Research. 2006;**84**(8):1645-1655. DOI: 10.1002/jnr.21065

[63] Bernabe A et al. Regulation of the Na+–dependent glutamate/aspartate transporter in rodent cerebellar astrocytes. Neurochemical Research. 2003;**28**(12):1843-1849 https://doi.org/10.1023/A%3A1026171724963

[64] Espinoza-Rojo M et al. Glast: Gene expression regulation by Phorbol esters. Neuroreport. 2000;**11**(12):2827-2832

[65] Guo D et al. Notch-1 regulates Akt signaling pathway and the expression of cell cycle regulatory proteins Cyclin D1, Cdk2 and P21 in T-all cell lines. Leukemia Research. 2009;**33**(5):678-685. DOI: 10.1016/j.leukres.2008.10.026

[66] Fitzgerald K et al. Ras pathway signals are required for notch-mediated oncogenesis. Oncogene. 2000;**19**(37):4191-4198. DOI: 10.1038/sj.onc.1203766

[67] Kim M et al. Protein kinase Cdelta negatively regulates Notch1-dependent transcription via a kinase-independent mechanism in vitro. Biochimica et Biophysica Acta. 2012;**1823**(2):387-397. DOI: 10.1016/j.bbamcr.2011.11.005

[68] Steinhart R et al. Pkcepsilon induces astrocytic differentiation of multipotential neural precursor cells. Glia. 2007;**55**(2):224-232. DOI: 10.1002/glia.20454

[69] Xu C et al. Morphine promotes astrocyte-preferential differentiation of mouse hippocampal progenitor cells via Pkcepsilon-dependent Erk activation and Trbp phosphorylation. Stem Cells. 2015;**33**(9):2762-2772. DOI: 10.1002/stem.2055

[70] Sjoqvist M et al. Pkczeta regulates notch receptor routing and activity in a notch signaling-dependent manner. Cell Research. 2014;**24**(4):433-450. DOI: 10.1038/cr.2014.34

[71] Guillem AM et al. Methylphenidate increases glutamate uptake in Bergmann glial cells. Neurochemical Research. 2015;**40**(11):2317-2324. DOI: 10.1007/s11064-015-1721-z

[72] Ohtsuka T et al. Hes1 and Hes5 as notch effectors in mammalian neuronal differentiation. The EMBO Journal. 1999;**18**(8):2196-2207. DOI: 10.1093/emboj/18.8.2196

[73] Lebkuechner I et al. Heterogeneity of notch signaling in astrocytes and the effects of Gfap and Vimentin deficiency. Journal of Neurochemistry. 2015;**135**(2):234-248. DOI: 10.1111/jnc.13213

[74] Endo Y et al. Bimodal functions of notch-mediated signaling are involved in neural crest formation during avian ectoderm development. Development. 2002;**129**(4):863-873

[75] Kwon C et al. Notch post-translationally regulates beta-catenin protein in stem and progenitor cells. Nature Cell Biology. 2011;**13**(10):1244-1251. DOI: 10.1038/ncb2313

[76] Ramain P et al. Novel notch alleles reveal a Deltex-dependent pathway repressing neural fate. Current Biology. 2001;**11**(22):1729-1738 https://doi.org/10.1016/S0960-9822(01)00562-0

[77] Endo Y et al. Deltex/Dtx mediates notch signaling in regulation of Bmp4 expression in cranial neural crest formation during avian development. Development, Growth & Differentiation. 2003;**45**(3):241-248. DOI: 10.1046/j.1524-4725.2003.693.x

[78] Kang JH et al. Protein kinase C (Pkc) isozyme-specific substrates and their design. Biotechnology Advances. 2012;**30**(6):1662-1672. DOI: 10.1016/j.biotechadv.2012.07.004

[79] Wu S et al. Targeting Glioma stem cells for therapy: Perspectives and challenges. Journal of Cell Science and Therapy. 2015;**6**(207). DOI: 10.4172/2157-7013.1000207

[80] Sugaya K. Stem cell biology in the study of pathological conditions. Neurodegenerative Diseases. 2010;**7**(1-3):84-87. DOI: 10.1159/000285512

[81] Kwak Y-D et al. Involvement of notch signaling pathway in amyloid precursor protein induced glial differentiation. European Journal of Pharmacology. 2011;**650**(1):18-27. DOI: 10.1016/j.ejphar.2010.09.015

[82] Yamamizu K et al. In vitro modeling of blood-brain barrier with human Ipsc-derived endothelial cells, pericytes, neurons, and astrocytes via notch signaling. Stem Cell Reports. 2017;**8**(3):634-647. DOI: 10.1016/j.stemcr.2017.01.023

[83] Wang K et al. Neuroprotective effects of Crocin against traumatic brain injury in mice: Involvement of notch signaling pathway. Neuroscience Letters. 2015;**591**:53-58. DOI: 10.1016/j.neulet.2015.02.016

[84] Wilhelmsson U et al. Astrocytes negatively regulate neurogenesis through the Jagged1-mediated notch pathway. Stem Cells. 2012;**30**(10):2320-2329. DOI: 10.1002/stem.1196

[85] Jurynczyk M et al. Inhibition of notch signaling enhances tissue repair in an animal model of multiple sclerosis. Journal of Neuroimmunology. 2005;**170**(1-2):3-10. DOI: 10.1016/j.jneuroim.2005.10.013

[86] Jurynczyk M et al. Overcoming failure to repair demyelination in Eae: Gamma-secretase inhibition of notch signaling. Journal of the Neurological Sciences. 2008;**265**(1-2):5-11. DOI: 10.1016/j.jns.2007.09.007

[87] Yang GS et al. Synergistic effect of mild hypothermia and the notch inhibitor Dapt against post stroke seizures. Biomedicine & Pharmacotherapy. 2017;**96**:675-684. DOI: 10.1016/j.biopha.2017.10.036

[88] Andersson ER et al. Therapeutic modulation of notch Signalling — Are we there yet? Nature Reviews Drug Discovery. 2014;**13**:357. DOI: 10.1038/nrd4252 https://www.nature.com/articles/nrd4252#supplementary-information

[89] Toritsuka M et al. Regulation of striatal dopamine responsiveness by notch/Rbp-J signaling. Translational Psychiatry. 2017;**7**:e1049. DOI: 10.1038/tp.2017.21 https://www.nature.com/articles/tp201721#supplementary-information

[90] Du J et al. Dner modulates the length, polarity and synaptogenesis of spiral ganglion neurons via the notch signaling pathway. Molecular Medicine Reports. 2017;**17**:2357-2365. DOI: 10.3892/mmr.2017.8115

Chapter 4

Pharmacological Studies with Specific Agonist and Antagonist of Animal iGluR on Root Growth in *Arabidopsis thaliana*

Shashi Kant Singh and Ing-Feng Chang

Additional information is available at the end of the chapter

http://dx.doi.org/10.5772/intechopen.72121

Abstract

Ionotropic glutamate receptors (iGluRs) are a group of proteins with a high degree of sequence homology. At least 20 type of putative ionotropic glutamate receptor (iGluR)-like channels have been identified in *Arabidopsis thaliana*. To uncover the role of iGluR-like channels in plant root growth, we used a comprehensive set of compounds known to alter iGluR channels in the neurons. We found that Arabidopsis root system is highly sensitive to these compounds. iGluR competitive antagonists 6-Cyano-7-nitroquinoxaline-2,3-dione (CNQX) or 6,7-dinitroquinoxaline-2,3-dione acted (DNQX) acts as a negative regulator of primary root and lateral root density. Continuous growth on antagonist also leads to impairment of root meristem size, which suggests that iGluR-like channels may play a role in meristem maintenance. However, application of iGluR agonists L-glutamate recovered Arabidopsis root growth. Taken together, these results suggest a correlation between the putative iGluR-like channel function and the alteration of root growth and development in the Arabidopsis roots.

Keywords: glutamate receptor, lateral root, Glu, calcium, DNQX, CNQX

1. Introduction

A mixture of organic and inorganic materials that makes uppermost layer of the earth in which plants grow is known as Soil. The parent mineral rock derives inorganic materials and is found in the form of sand, silt and clay. However, organic materials come from dead and decayed parts of bacteria, fungi, algae, protozoa and soil animals such as nematodes, earthworms, beetles and termites. The inorganic nitrogen dissolved in soil is vital for nutritional requirements of plants, and it can be directly used in the synthesis of amino acids, peptides and proteins [1]. Plants absorb organic nitrogen from soil in the form of free amino acids [2, 3], which is derived mainly from decomposed organic matter and exudates produced by bacteria, fungus and living plants roots [4–9].

Among the 20 common amino acids, the six amino acids (glutamic acid, glutamine, aspartic acid, asparagine, alanine and histidine) are mainly dominated in the soil, and they cover approximately 80% of the total soil amino acid pool [10–12].

An agonist is an inducing ligand that can bind to and induce channel-linked receptors. On the contrary, antagonist is a type of receptor ligand that can block the agonist-mediated responses. Since ionotropic glutamate receptors (iGluRs) are ligand-gated ion channels, binding of L-glutamate (Glu) will open gates and increase ions conductance. However, both agonists and antagonists of iGluRs share structural similarity with glutamate and bind to iGluRs at the same site where Glu binds [13]. Interestingly, it has been observed that major amino acids (glutamate, glycine, alanine, serine, asparagine, and cysteine) present in the rhizosphere are strong agonist for iGlurRs [14].

Previous studies indicate that plant GLRs are functional, and involved in various functions, such as photosynthesis [15, 16], abiotic stress [17, 18], as C/N balance [19], plant-pathogen interaction [20, 21], root morphogenesis [22–24], pollen tube growth [25] and regulate cellular calcium homeostasis [14, 20, 26–29]. Among studies with various cell types in plants, it was found that Glu induces intracellular Ca^{2+} current. Glu-induced rise in the intracellular Ca^{2+} level can be inhibited by the use of iGluRs antagonists, which are quinoxalinediones, 6,7-dinitroquinoxaline-2,3-dione (DNQX) and 6-cyano-7-nitroquinoxaline-2,3-dione (CNQX) [18, 27, 30]. Therefore, it was proposed that glutamate receptors (GLRs) can contribute to the network of Ca^{2+} signaling pathways in plant cells [16]. *Atglr1.2* knock-out mutant plants displayed abnormalities in pollen growth [25]. Further, Analysis of *Arabidopsis* GLR mutant, *atglr3.6*, reveals a major role of the plant GLRs in the regulation of plant root development [24]. As a signaling molecule, glutamate is regarded to be the major neurotransmitter in the mammalian central nervous system. The application of exogenous Glu can also alter root phenotype [31, 32], indicating a role for GLR signaling in plants. Additionally, MEKK pathways can alter the glutamate sensitivity at the root tip suggesting for a glutamate signaling pathway in plants [33, 34].

These days pharmacology-based functional study of ionotropic glutamate receptors in plants has become very popular and useful approach [17, 18, 27, 32, 35–37]. We used comprehensive set of compounds that have been found to contain a strong ability to modulate the activity of mammalian iGluRs. In the present study, we introduced Glu to study the possible role of plant GLRs in root development. To minimize the chance of multiple effects of Glu, we also used artificial agonists (NMDA and AMPA) and competitive antagonists (DNQX and CNQX) to the glutamate binding site on receptors. In animals, these artificial agonists and antagonists are reported only for specific effects via their impact on iGluR activities [38]. In our pharmacological-based study, we investigate how glutamate and iGluRs antagonists directly affect plant root growth and development.

http://dx.doi.org/10.5772/intechopen.72121

2. Materials and methods

2.1. Plant materials and growth conditions

Arabidopsis thaliana (Col-0) seedlings were used in different analyses on root development. All seed germination treatments were carried out at same half-strength Murashige and Skoog (MS) medium [39] at constant pH 5.8. The root elongation under various treatments was quantified using ImageJ program (http://rsb.info.nih.gov/ij/).

2.2. Chemicals

L-aspartic acid (Sigma, USA), L-glutamic acid, monosodium salt (Sigma, USA), N-Methyl-D-aspartate (NMDA; Sigma, USA), and 2-amino-3-(5-methyl-3-oxo-1,2- oxazol-4-yl) propanoic acid (AMPA; Sigma, USA) were dissolved in water, adjusted to pH 5.8 and filter sterilized. Both receptor antagonists, 6,7-dinitroquinoxaline-2,3-dione (DNQX; Sigma, USA) and 6-cyano-7-nitroquinoxaline-2,3-dione (CNQX; Tocris, USA) were dissolved in organic solvent Dimethyl sulfoxide (DMSO) (Sigma, USA). All treatments were used with variable concentrations as indicated in the figure legends. In order to study the role of Glu in auxin balance inside the root cells, we used a synthetic auxin Naphthaleneacetic acid (NAA, Sigma) and a polar auxin transport inhibitor NPA (1-N-Naphthylphthalamic acid, Sigma) for treatments.

2.3. Seed sterilization

Prior to germination at growth media, seeds were first surface-sterilized in sodium hypochlorite in active chlorine. Sterilization was carried out in a hood cabinet, and aliquots of seeds were placed in Eppendorf tubes and treated with active chlorine for 1–2 h.

2.4. Plant growth condition

Arabidopsis seedlings for analysis were grown in sterile petri dishes using half strength MS medium and the plate was sealed using Micropore TM tape. After this, seeds were stratified in the dark at 4°C for 2–3 days to synchronize germination. Plates were then transferred to a growth chamber at illumination of 120–150 μmol/m^2 s continuous light and at temperature 22–23°C.

2.5. Laser scanning and light microscopy

Confocal microscopy was performed using a Zeiss LSM510 META Confocal Imaging System (USA). To observe the apical root meristem through confocal microscopy, roots were counterstained in propidium iodide (PI, Sigma) (10 μM) for 2–3 min, rinsed, mounted in dH_2O. Images were obtained by excitation with the Kr/Ar 488-nm laser line and emission was detected with a band-pass 500–550 nm filter.

2.6. Statistical analysis

Each experiment was repeated at least three times. Values are expressed as mean ± SD. The statistical significance was analyzed using Student's *t*-test analysis.

3. Results

3.1. iGluR agonists and antagonists alter root growth in Arabidopsis

We used a comprehensive set of compounds that have been found to modulate iGluRs. All treatments were performed with half strength of MS media [39] at a constant pH 5.8. The presence these compounds was observed to have a marked effect on root architecture of Arabidopsis. Both Glu and NMDA treatments had a stimulatory effect on primary root length (PRL) as well as lateral root density (LRD) in wild-type plants as compared to the non-treated plants. However, up to 10 days, AMPA showed a minor effect on root growth, but afterward, AMPA addition also nearly restored root growth of wild-type plants, making it visually indistinguishable from that of NMDA-treated plants (**Figure 1A** and **B**). These results indicated that glutamate receptor agonists likely interact with signaling pathways to control root growth in plants. Further, to test whether root growth was specific to natural iGluR ligands (Glu), we used another kind of neurotransmitter amino acid L-aspartate (Asp) [40]. Interestingly, after 12 days of growth, Asp treatment showed modest activity at inhibiting root growth and failed to increase lateral root formation when supplied at the same concentrations as Glu (**Figure 1A** and **B**). These results indicate that Glu and Asp have different activity in Arabidopsis root growth modulation and that the effects of Glu on root development are likely due to a specific effect of Glu rather than as a consequence of acidic behavior of amino acids.

To determine more closely the effects of plant iGluR-like receptor on the architecture of the Arabidopsis root system, wild-type Arabidopsis seedlings were germinated and grown on vertically oriented agar plates containing half strength MS medium supplemented with iGluR antagonists (DNQX and CNQX) alone or in combination of antagonists with Glu. As expected, our results show that both DNQX and CNQX drastically reduced root growth, and induced approximately similar kind of effects on root growth (**Figure 1C** and **D**). It was seen that the PRL approximately reduced by 64.65% and 69.24% and LRD by 76.1% and 76.55% (respectively for DNQX and CNQX treatment) (**Figure 1C** and **D**). To observe the effect of agonist and antagonist treatment together, we used naturally occurring agonist, Glu, to compete with DNQX and CNQX inhibitory actions [41]. It was observed that the external supplement of Glu (at 0.5 mM) successfully recovered the reduced root growth (both PRL and LRD) (**Figure 1C** and **D**). In summary, root growth was promoted by iGluR agonists, and use of iGluR antagonists (CNQX and DNQX) drastically reduced root growth and then, again subsequently recovered by addition of Glu suggesting molecular correlation. Since, these comprehensive set of compounds are called the great modulator of iGluRs in mammalian cells, our results suggested the involvement of Arabidopsis iGluR-like channel in root development.

http://dx.doi.org/10.5772/intechopen.72121

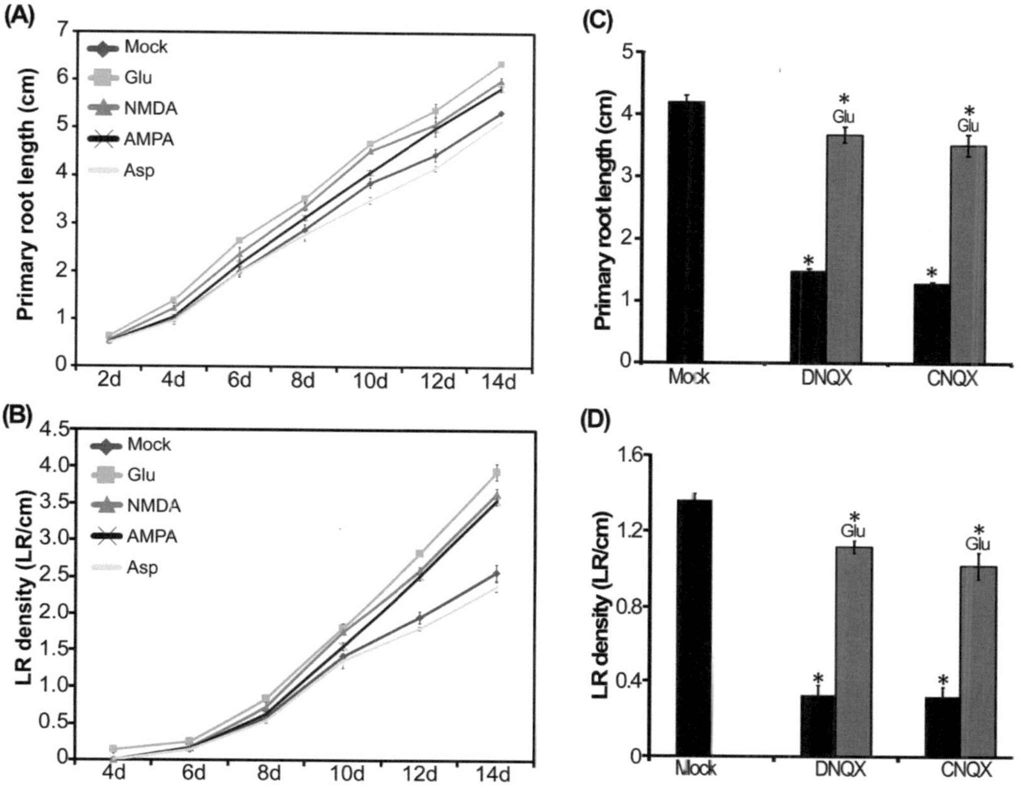

Figure 1. Variable effects of animal iGluR effector compounds on *Arabidopsis thaliana* root development. Arabidopsis (wild-type, Col-0 ecotype) seedlings were germinated on half strength of MS medium (MS/2, [39]) supplemented with 1% of sucrose and agar. Immediately after germination, different treatments were done in MS/2 basal media adjusted to pH 5.8 with NaOH. Time course for agonist treatments response in days 2–14 of longitudinal primary root growth (A) and LR density (B) represented as LRs per centimeter primary root of Col-0 after incubation with 0.5 mM of each glutamate (Glu), NMDA, AMPA and aspartate (Asp) individually. Antagonist's treatments were done in MS/2 basal media but control seedlings (Mock) were grown with equal volume of solvent (DMSO) as in DNQX (1 mM) and CNQX (1 mM) treated seedlings. Comparison of root growth under antagonist given alone (1 mM) or together in the treatment of 0.5 mM Glu. Root length (C) and LR density (D) of 11-day-old Col-0 seedlings. Values represent the mean of 15–18 measurements in triplicate and error bars represent ±SD. The statistical analysis were performed by Student's *t*-test ($P < 0.005$) indicated by asterisks.

3.2. Short-root growth in antagonist treated wild-type roots is contributed by reduced root meristem size

Previously we concluded that the glutamate receptor signaling may be involved in regulatory mechanisms in the control of root growth, indicating an essential role for plant GLRs in root meristem maintenance Therefore we analyzed cell division and meristem size among wild-type and antagonist-treated wild-type roots at different growth duration (4 and 6 days). However, since treatments of both antagonists induced similar kind of inhibitory effect on root growth, and thus we selected only one antagonist (DNQX) for further studies.

Interestingly, we observed that antagonist-treated wild-type root illustrated a smaller meristem size compared to wild-type (**Figure 2A** and **B**). Simultaneously, the number of meristematic epidermal cells (in a single file) was also significantly reduced in both 4 and 6-day-old roots of DNQX-treated wild-type plants (**Figure 2C**). Reduced meristem-enriched tissues in DNQX treated roots showed a putative vital contribution of putative *AtGLR* signaling in Arabidopsis root development.

QC surrounded with stem cells are pivotal in cell proliferation and meristem maintenance in root [42]. Thus we investigated the possibility of deformity in the stem cell niche which may result in impaired root growth after antagonist treatment. In confocal sections of propidium iodide (PI) stained roots (**Figure 3A** and **B**), we observed that in comparison to wild-type (four-celled QC), DNQX-treated wild-type roots were characterized by small dislocated columella cells with complicated-cellular-patterns. Altered columella root cap cells can also be

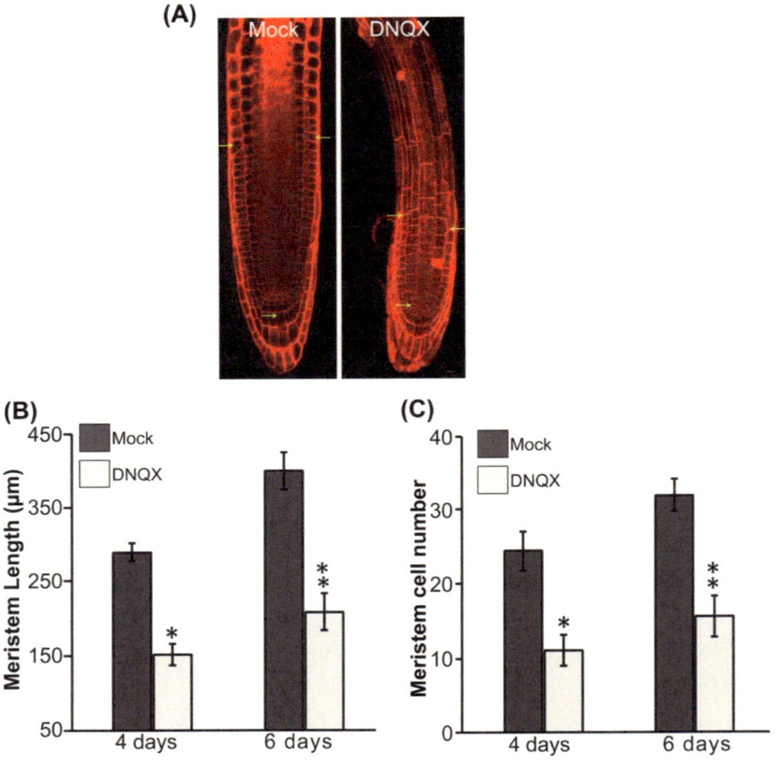

Figure 2. Putative AtGLR regulates meristematic activity in primary-root apical meristem. (A) Confocal microscopic images of PI-stained 4-day-old wild-type and DNQX treated wild-type root. The border of root apical meristem is indicated by arrows in PI-stained roots. The longitudinal distance between the quiescent center (QC, marked in lower arrow) and the first elongating cell is correspond to the root meristem length (B) and the number of meristematic epidermal cells in single file of cells in wild-type and DNQX treated wild-type root at various time points (4 and 6-day-old seedling) (C). Error bars represent SE ($n > 15$). Statistical significance in compared with wild-type were analyzed by Student's *t*-test ($P < 0.005$).

observed by Lugol staining of starch granule [43]. We found that DNQX treatment in wild-type approximately abolished the starch grains from amyloplast (**Figure 3C** and **D**).

3.3. Externally supplied Glu can rescue the EGTA-inhibited root phenotypes

There are many studies which showed that Arabidopsis AtGLRs engage in calcium homeostasis [27, 28, 30]. We investigated whether the induced root growth in Glu-treated seedlings was dependent on Ca^{2+}. Various concentrations of EGTA (a Ca^{2+} chelator) was added to MS/2 supplemented with 0.5 mM Glu. At both concentrations of EGTA (0.5 and 1.0 mM), root elongation was drastically inhibited in wild-type seedlings. However, supplement of external Glu partially recovered root growth inhibited by low amount of EGTA (**Figure 4**). Collectively, these data suggest a role for Ca^{2+} in AtGLRs signaling to control root growth.

Auxin has been recognized as a key regulator in root development [44, 45]. NPA is a drug that known for inhibition of polar auxin transport. An induction of cytosolic Ca^{2+} was observed after auxin application, indicating a strong correlations between Ca^{2+} and auxin signaling. Therefore, we investigated whether the higher root growth observed in the Glu-treated seedlings is linked to the auxin and calcium. To elucidate this, we investigated whether Glu and $CaCl_2$ are able to minimize the negative effect of NPA on Arabidopsis root growth. Interestingly, applications of Glu and $CaCl_2$ to NPA-treated wild-type seedling had restored the number of LR (**Figure 5A** and **B**).

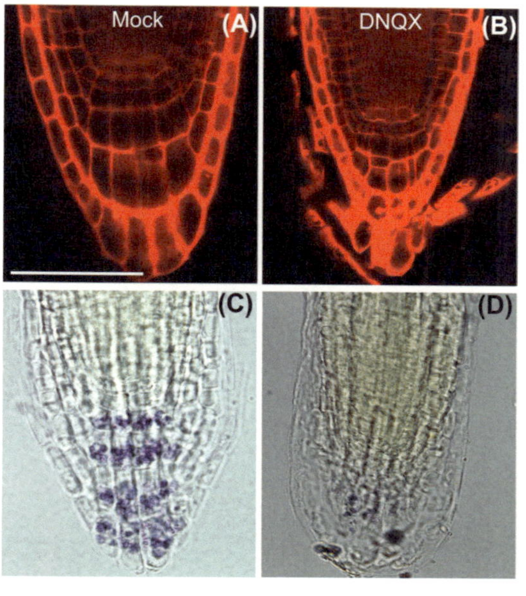

Figure 3. Putative AtGLR regulates meristematic activity in primary-root apical meristem. Statistical significance in compared with wild-type were analyzed by Student's *t*-test ($P < 0.005$), indicated by asterisk. (A–B) Confocal images of 4-day-old PI-stained wild-type and DNQX treated wild-type roots. Columella cells have abnormal cell divisions in DNQX treated wild-type roots. Wild-type and DNQX treated wild-type roots in Lugol staining (C–D). Scale bar: 100 μm.

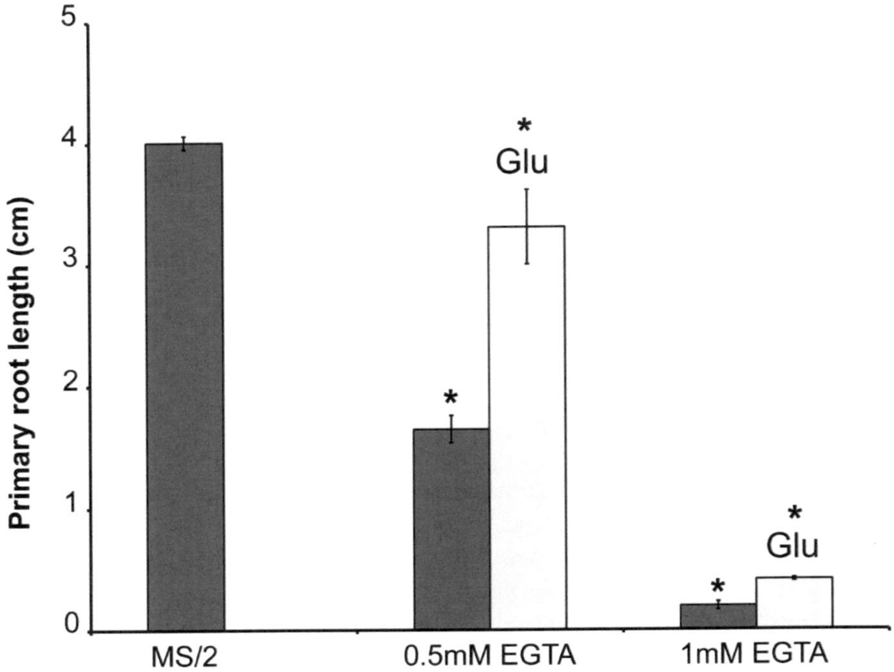

Figure 4. Ca^{2+}-dependent growth phenotypes of EGTA treated wild-type root seedlings. Putative ligand Glu can overcome reduced root growth by low amount of EGTA. Root phenotype of the 10-day-old wild-type seedlings under the different treatments. Supplement of 0.5 mM Glu successfully recovered the primary root growth which was reduced by 0.5 mM and 1 mM EGTA. The data presented are averages of three biological replicates. Asterisks represent statistical difference analyzed with a Student's *t*-test; $P < 0.005$, $n = 15$.

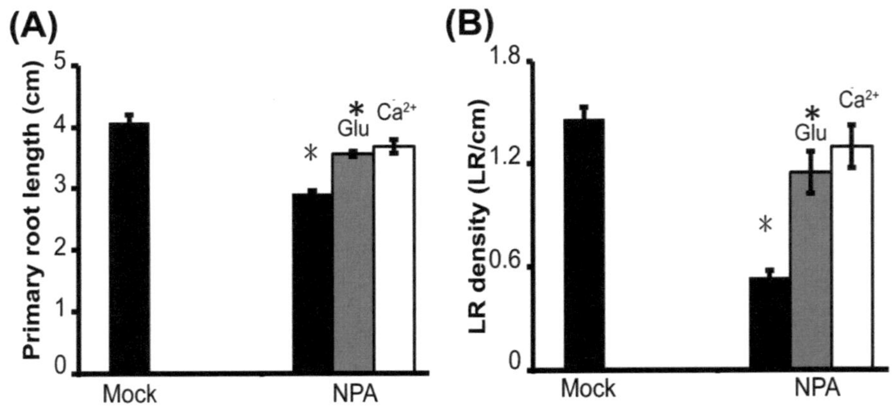

Figure 5. Reduced root growth shown by NPA-treated wild-type roots can be rescued by the externally supplied Glu. Recovery of arrested root growth suggest the role of auxin. Application 1-N-Naphthylphthalamic acid (NPA) caused arrest of root growth. However, exogenous application of Glu and Ca^{2+} (0.5 mM) to NPA-treated root is successfully minimized the NPA effect (A and B). Asterisks represent statistical difference analyzed with a Student's *t*-test; $P < 0.005$, $n = 15$.

4. Discussion

4.1. Effect of glutamate treatment on root growth

Root plays pivotal role in plant life as it is crucial for nutrient and water absorption. In *Arabidopsis thaliana*, a total of 20 types of AtGLR subunits have been identified. They have significantly high sequence similarity with animal iGluR-like channels [46]. Probably due to phylogenetically conserved amino acid sequences, they may have a high potential for functional redundancy. Using specific drugs that alter the channel activities is a key to study the function of iGluR-like channels in Arabidopsis [21]. We used Glu, (a neurotransmitter), and other set of compounds known to agonize (activate) (NMDA and AMAP) and antagonize (deactivate) (DNQX and CNQX) the iGluR channels in mammalian cells. The use of broader set of drugs would allowed us to observe the specific effects related to Glu and iGluR-like channels in root cells. We observed that the application of these drugs potentially modulate the Arabidopsis root architectures indicating an importance for AtGLRs in root development. We observed that the application of iGluR agonists, Glu and NMDA were promoting root growth. In other studies it has also been reported that Glu could act as a root growth modifier [32, 47, 48]. Because Glu is an acidic amino acid which can cause low pH-induced toxicity (acidic), which could reduce root growth [31, 32, 48], we performed all experiments on constant pH range from 5.7 to 5.8 designed for plant tissue culture medium. Our result showing correlation with other evidences which have been proved that plants possess Glu-activated ion channels like iGluRs [30, 35, 36]. More specifically, NMDA-like iGluR receptors are also predicted in plants [27, 49]. Ammonium ion is a key form of inorganic nitrogen. Organic nitrogen compounds (amino acids, nucleic acids *etc.*) are derived from NH_4^+ [50]. The assimilation of NH_4^+ into Glu is the crucial step in amino acid synthesis and nitrogen metabolism [51]. Glu is directly involved chlorophyll synthesis in developing leaves [52]. Although it cannot be ruled out that Glu metabolism plays an important part in plant nitrogen assimilation and its regulation, increasing evidence suggests signaling properties of Glu in animals may also develop in plant [53].

The specificity of Glu to promote root development is individual. We used another kind of amino acid neurotransmitter, aspartate (Asp). Unlike Glu, it failed to induce root growth, showing Glu signaling in root development is highly specific [19]. Both DNQX and CNQX are the potent competitive AMPA/kainate glutamate receptor antagonists [38, 54]. We reported that iGluR antagonists have drastic effect on root growth. In animals they are known to block the ionotropic glutamate receptors very precisely [55]. Moreover, some studies in plants also have defined that animal iGluR antagonist are capable of changing the ion activity inside the cells and hence the phenotypes [16, 19, 21, 35, 56]. More interestingly, additional supply of Glu is able to counter the negative effect of each antagonist, suggesting a strong evidence of the existence of functional glutamate receptors in plant root development [17, 19, 20, 37, 56]. Similar evidence is also reported. Glu and Gly successfully revert back the effect of DNQX on Arabidopsis hypocotyl growth [27].

4.2. Root meristematic activity

In Arabidopsis, root meristem develops from a stem-cell niche situated at the apical part of the root [57, 58]. Glutamate Receptor–Like protein (GLR3.1) has been described to be essential for meristematic activity in roots [22]. The roots grown by antagonist treatment significantly reduced meristematic cell number, and hence a contraction of meristem size was also observed. These observations certainly showed a correlation with less root growth under antagonist treatment [59]. The role of quiescent center (QC) is vital in the maintenance of root meristem [58, 60]. The majority of cells in the root meristem develop from stem cells which are derived from QC. In confocal microscopic analysis, antagonist treated-root showed a major change in QC organization which may resulted in less developed root meristem [61]. Numerous sedimented starch-filled amyloplasts in the root cap are distinguishing of columella cells [62]. In our study it was observed that columella cells of antagonist treated-roots possessed of defective amyloplasts in Lugol staining [63]. Therefore short root phenotype is highly consistence with defected organization of the root cap and QC [42, 64, 65].

4.3. Glutamate and calcium in root growth

The iGluR is known to be a Ca^{2+} permeable channel [66]. Many studies revealed that Arabidopsis AtGLR induces Ca^{2+} current upon activation by Glu [27, 30, 67]. We investigated whether the putative agonist and antagonist treatments alter the $[Ca^{2+}]$cyt level in roots. EGTA is a well-known Ca^{2+}-chelating agents [68]. In our study, application of EGTA shows a strong inhibition in root growth. Interestingly, however when Glu was introduced in same media, root growth was resumed. The presence of EGTA allows low availability of Ca^{2+} in free space. Animal cells and plant cells are similar in that they are both use endoplasmic reticulum (ER) as a calcium storage. Glutamate receptors are also reported to localized in ER [22, 69]. In animals, Glu-induced intracellular calcium levels through endoplasmic reticulum is reported [69]. However, application of Glu may lead to more activation of putative AtGLRs that allow more Ca^{2+} release to cytoplasm from endomembrane system which might play a role to recover the root growth. Calcium is key regulator of root growth [70, 71]. Previous report has also found that roots in EGTA containing media failed to grow toward gravity but it could be recovered by extra Ca^{2+} supply [72]. Furthermore, as we have discussed before that application of DNQX and CNQX reduced root apical meristem and hence also root growth, but application external Ca^{2+} could resume root growth. These results suggest a role of AtGLRs in Arabidopsis root development.

4.4. Glutamate signaling and polar auxin transport in roots

Expressions of *AtGLR* genes inside the root tissue give strong evidence that these receptors have vital role [46, 73]. Recent studies on chimeric and other plant iGLRs provided evidence for Ca^{2+} permeability across membranes. We have also found that the *glr3.6-1* mutant showed altered cytosolic calcium levels in root cells [24]. Calcium and auxin work together in many aspects of cellular processes. A similar effect has been observed in different studies in response to calcium-chelating agents. Dela Fuente and Leopold (1973) showed that basipetal transport of auxin is depressed by EDTA treatment and that subsequent addition of Ca^{2+} restores auxin transport in roots [74]. Root bend toward a calcium-containing agar block versus an agar block with the calcium-chelating agent EGTA, suggesting that auxin transport is regulated by local $[Ca^{2+}]_{cyt}$ levels [72]. NPA is a potent polar auxin transport inhibitor, which can highly reduce the lateral root emergence [75–77]. Supplement of Glu together with NPA (1-N-Naphthylphthalamic acid) (at 0.5 mM) showed approximately close root phenotype to the control seedlings. Addition of Glu in intact roots directly may induce Ca^{2+} which may lead to enhanced auxin transport and hence the suppressed negative effect of NPA Possibly application of Glu can enhance the auxin supply to other deserved root cells rather than showing competition with NPA blockage.

5. Conclusion

In this study, we applied a comprehensive set of compounds to study how these compounds affect Arabidopsis root growth. Arabidopsis root system is highly sensitive to these compounds known to alter the iGluR channels. Both Glu and NMDA promote the primary root growth and lateral root density in Arabidopsis. On the other hand, iGluR antagonists drastically reduced root growth at both parameters. Exogenous application of Glu successfully rescued reduced root phenotype inhibited by EGTA. Moreover, root growth reduced by polar auxin transport inhibitor NPA, could be rescued by Glu and $CaCl_2$. As for AtGLRs function, although the mechanisms are not yet clear, the results presented provide evidence in support of a role of AtGLRs in regulating Arabidopsis root development.

Acknowledgements

This work was supported by grants from Ministry of Science and Technology, Taiwan (MOST# 104-2311-B-002-034, MOST#106-2311-B-002-014, and MOST#106-2313-B-002-004). We thank TechComm (College of Life Science, NTU, Taiwan) for very helpful technical assistance.

Author details

Shashi Kant Singh[1] and Ing-Feng Chang[1,2,3]*

*Address all correspondence to: ifchang@ntu.edu.tw

1 Institute of Plant Biology, National Taiwan University, Taipei, Taiwan

2 Department of Life Science, National Taiwan University, Taipei, Taiwan

3 Genome and Systems Biology Degree Program, National Taiwan University and Academia Sinica, Taipei, Taiwan

References

[1] Lipson D, Nasholm T. The unexpected versatility of plants: Organic nitrogen use and availability in terrestrial ecosystems. Oecologia. 2001;**128**:305-316

[2] Kielland K. Amino acid absorption by arctic plants: Implications for plant nutrition and nitrogen cycling. Ecology. 1994;**75**:2373-2383

[3] Nordin A, Uggla C, Nasholm T. Nitrogen forms in bark, wood and foliage of nitrogen-fertilized *Pinus sylvestris*. Tree Physiology. 2001;**21**:59-64

[4] Barzana G, Aroca R, Bienert GP, Chaumont F, Ruiz-Lozano JM. New insights into the regulation of aquaporins by the arbuscular mycorrhizal symbiosis in maize plants under drought stress and possible implications for plant performance. Molecular Plant-Microbe Interactions. 2014;**27**:349-363

[5] Butler JL, Williams MA, Bottomley PJ, Myrold DD. Microbial community dynamics associated with rhizosphere carbon flow. Applied and Environmental Microbiology. 2003;**69**:6793-6800

[6] Dennis PG, Miller AJ, Hirsch PR. Are root exudates more important than other sources of rhizodeposits in structuring rhizosphere bacterial communities? FEMS Microbiology Ecology. 2010;**72**:313-327

[7] Ramos C, Licht TR, Sternberg C, Krogfelt KA, Molin S. Monitoring bacterial growth activity in biofilms from laboratory flow chambers, plant rhizosphere, and animal intestine. Methods in Enzymology. 2001;**337**:21-42

[8] Walder F, Brule D, Koegel S, Wiemken A, Boller T, Courty PE. Plant phosphorus acquisition in a common mycorrhizal network: Regulation of phosphate transporter genes of the Pht1 family in sorghum and flax. The New Phytologist. 2015;**205**:1632-1645

[9] Weintraub MN, Scott-Denton LE, Schmidt SK, Monson RK. The effects of tree rhizodeposition on soil exoenzyme activity, dissolved organic carbon, and nutrient availability in a subalpine forest ecosystem. Oecologia. 2007;**154**:327-338

[10] Bremner JM. The amino-acid composition of the protein material in soil. The Biochemical Journal. 1950;**47**:538-542

[11] Martens DA, Loeffelmann KL. Soil amino acid composition quantified by acid hydrolysis and anion chromatography-pulsed amperometry. Journal of Agricultural and Food Chemistry. 2003;**51**:6521-6529

[12] Nancy RW. Soil amino acid composition across a boreal forest successional sequence. Soil Biology & Biochemistry. 2009;**41**:1210-1220

[13] Schwartz EA, Tachibana M. Electrophysiology of glutamate and sodium co-transport in a glial cell of the salamander retina. The Journal of Physiology. 1990;**426**:43-80

[14] Qi Z, Stephens NR, Spalding EP. Calcium entry mediated by GLR3.3, an Arabidopsis glutamate receptor with a broad agonist profile. Plant Physiology. 2006;**142**:963-971

[15] Teardo E, Formentin E, Segalla A, Giacometti GM, Marin O, Zanetti M, Lo Schiavo F, Zoratti M, Szabo I. Dual localization of plant glutamate receptor AtGLR3.4 to plastids and plasma membrane. Biochimica et Biophysica Acta. 2011;**1807**:359-367

[16] Teardo E, Segalla A, Formentin E, Zanetti M, Marin O, Giacometti GM, Lo Schiavo F, Zoratti M, Szabo I. Characterization of a plant glutamate receptor activity. Cellular Physiology and Biochemistry. 2010;**26**:253-262

[17] Kang J, Mehta S, Turano FJ. The putative glutamate receptor 1.1 (AtGLR1.1) in *Arabidopsis thaliana* regulates abscisic acid biosynthesis and signaling to control development and water loss. Plant & Cell Physiology. 2004;**45**:1380-1389

[18] Meyerhoff O, Muller K, Roelfsema MR, Latz A, Lacombe B, Hedrich R, Dietrich P, Becker D. AtGLR3.4, a glutamate receptor channel-like gene is sensitive to touch and cold. Planta. 2005;**222**:418-427

[19] Kang J, Turano FJ. The putative glutamate receptor 1.1 (AtGLR1.1) functions as a regulator of carbon and nitrogen metabolism in *Arabidopsis thaliana*. Proceedings of the National Academy of Sciences of the United States of America. 2003;**100**:6872-6877

[20] Kang S, Kim HB, Lee H, Choi JY, Heu S, Oh CJ, Kwon SI, An CS. Overexpression in Arabidopsis of a plasma membrane-targeting glutamate receptor from small radish increases glutamate-mediated Ca^{2+} influx and delays fungal infection. Molecules and Cells. 2006;**21**:418-427

[21] Kwaaitaal M, Huisman R, Maintz J, Reinstadler A, Panstruga R. Ionotropic glutamate receptor (iGluR)-like channels mediate MAMP-induced calcium influx in *Arabidopsis thaliana*. The Biochemical Journal. 2011;**440**:355-365

[22] Li J, Zhu S, Song X, Shen Y, Chen H, Yu J, Yi K, Liu Y, Karplus VJ, Wu P, Deng XW. A rice glutamate receptor-like gene is critical for the division and survival of individual cells in the root apical meristem. Plant Cell. 2006;**18**:340-349

[23] Miller ND, Durham Brooks TL, Assadi AH, Spalding EP. Detection of a gravitropism phenotype in glutamate receptor-like 3.3 mutants of *Arabidopsis thaliana* using machine vision and computation. Genetics. 2010;**186**:585-593

[24] Singh SK, Chien CT, Chang IF. The Arabidopsis glutamate receptor-like gene GLR3.6 controls root development by repressing the Kip-related protein gene KRP4. Journal of Experimental Botany. 2016;**67**:1853-1869

[25] Michard E, Lima PT, Borges F, Silva AC, Portes MT, Carvalho JE, Gilliham M, Liu LH, Obermeyer G, Feijo JA. Glutamate receptor-like genes form Ca^{2+} channels in pollen tubes and are regulated by pistil D-serine. Science. 2011;**332**:434-437

[26] Cho D, Kim SA, Murata Y, Lee S, Jae SK, Nam HG, Kwak JM. De-regulated expression of the plant glutamate receptor homolog AtGLR3.1 impairs long-term Ca^{2+}-programmed stomatal closure. The Plant Journal. 2009;**58**:437-449

[27] Dubos C, Huggins D, Grant GH, Knight MR, Campbell MM. A role for glycine in the gating of plant NMDA-like receptors. The Plant Journal. 2003;**35**:800-810

[28] Kim SA, Kwak JM, Jae SK, Wang MH, Nam HG. Overexpression of the AtGluR2 gene encoding an Arabidopsis homolog of mammalian glutamate receptors impairs calcium utilization and sensitivity to ionic stress in transgenic plants. Plant & Cell Physiology. 2001;**42**:74-84

[29] Vincill ED, Bieck AM, Spalding EP. Ca(2+) conduction by an amino acid-gated ion channel related to glutamate receptors. Plant Physiology. 2012;**159**:40-46

[30] Dennison KL, Spalding EP. Glutamate-gated calcium fluxes in Arabidopsis. Plant Physiology. 2000;**124**:1511-1514

[31] Kim TH, Kim EC, Kim SW, Lee HS, Choi DW. Exogenous glutamate inhibits the root growth and increases the glutamine content in *Arabidopsis thaliana*. Journal of Plant Biology. 2010;**53**:45-51

[32] Walch-Liu P, Forde BG. L-Glutamate as a novel modifier of root growth and branching: What's the sensor? Plant Signaling & Behavior. 2007;**2**:284-286

[33] Forde BG. Glutamate signalling in roots. Journal of Experimental Botany. 2014;**65**:779-787

[34] Forde BG, Cutler SR, Zaman N, Krysan PJ. Glutamate signalling via a MEKK1 kinase-dependent pathway induces changes in Arabidopsis root architecture. The Plant Journal. 2013;**75**:1-10

[35] Brenner ED, Martinez-Barboza N, Clark AP, Liang QS, Stevenson DW, Coruzzi GM. Arabidopsis mutants resistant to S(+)-beta-methyl-alpha, beta-diaminopropionic acid, a cycad-derived glutamate receptor agonist. Plant Physiology. 2000;**124**:1615-1624

[36] Dubos C, Willment J, Huggins D, Grant GH, Campbell MM. Kanamycin reveals the role played by glutamate receptors in shaping plant resource allocation. The Plant Journal. 2005;**43**:348-355

[37] Sivaguru M, Pike S, Gassmann W, Baskin TI. Aluminum rapidly depolymerizes cortical microtubules and depolarizes the plasma membrane: Evidence that these responses are mediated by a glutamate receptor. Plant & Cell Physiology. 2003;**44**:667-675

[38] Alford S, Grillner S. CNQX and DNQX block non-NMDA synaptic transmission but not NMDA-evoked locomotion in lamprey spinal cord. Brain Research. 1990;**506**:297-302

[39] Murashige T, Skoog F. A revised medium for rapid growth and bioassays with tobacco tissue cultures. Plant Physiology. 1962;**15**:473-497

[40] Cavallero A, Marte A, Fedele E. L-aspartate as an amino acid neurotransmitter: Mechanisms of the depolarization-induced release from cerebrocortical synaptosomes. Journal of Neurochemistry. 2009;**110**:924-934

[41] Geoffroy M, Lambolez B, Audinat E, Hamon B, Crepel F, Rossier J, Kado RT. Reduction of desensitization of a glutamate ionotropic receptor by antagonists. Molecular Pharmacology. 1991;**39**:587-591

[42] van den Berg C, Willemsen V, Hendriks G, Weisbeek P, Scheres B. Short-range control of cell differentiation in the Arabidopsis root meristem. Nature. 1997;**390**:287-289

[43] Qin C, Yi KK, Wu P. Ammonium affects cell viability to inhibit root growth in Arabidopsis. Journal of Zhejiang University. Science. B. 2011;**12**:477-484

[44] Laskowski MJ, Williams ME, Nusbaum HC, Sussex IM. Formation of lateral root meristems is a two-stage process. Development. 1995;**121**:3303-3310

[45] Overvoorde P, Fukaki H, Beeckman T. Auxin control of root development. Cold Spring Harbor Perspectives in Biology. 2010;**2**:a001537

[46] Chiu JC, Brenner ED, DeSalle R, Nitabach MN, Holmes TC, Coruzzi GM. Phylogenetic and expression analysis of the glutamate-receptor-like gene family in *Arabidopsis thaliana*. Molecular Biology and Evolution. 2002;**19**:1066-1082

[47] Walch-Liu P, Forde BG. Nitrate signalling mediated by the NRT1.1 nitrate transporter antagonises L-glutamate-induced changes in root architecture. The Plant Journal. 2008;**54**:820-828

[48] Walch-Liu P, Liu LH, Remans T, Tester M, Forde BG. Evidence that L-glutamate can act as an exogenous signal to modulate root growth and branching in *Arabidopsis thaliana*. Plant & Cell Physiology. 2006;**47**:1045-1057

[49] Chiu J, DeSalle R, Lam HM, Meisel L, Coruzzi G. Molecular evolution of glutamate receptors: A primitive signaling mechanism that existed before plants and animals diverged. Molecular Biology and Evolution. 1999;**16**:826-838

[50] Storey R, Beevers L. Enzymology of glutamine metabolism related to senescence and seed development in the pea (*Pisum sativum* L.). Plant Physiology. 1978;**61**:494-500

[51] Suzuki A, Knaff DB. Glutamate synthase: Structural, mechanistic and regulatory properties, and role in the amino acid metabolism. Photosynthesis Research. 2005;**83**:191-217

[52] Yaronskaya E, Vershilovskaya I, Poers Y, Alawady AE, Averina N, Grimm B. Cytokinin effects on tetrapyrrole biosynthesis and photosynthetic activity in barley seedlings. Planta. 2006;**224**:700-709

[53] Forde BG, Lea PJ. Glutamate in plants: Metabolism, regulation, and signalling. Journal of Experimental Botany. 2007;**58**:2339-2358

[54] Lee SH, Govindaiah G, Cox CL. Selective excitatory actions of DNQX and CNQX in rat thalamic neurons. Journal of Neurophysiology. 2010;**103**:1728-1734

[55] Bessho Y, Nakanishi S, Nawa H. Glutamate receptor agonists enhance the expression of BDNF mRNA in cultured cerebellar granule cells. Brain Research. Molecular Brain Research. 1993;**18**:201-208

[56] Lam HM, Chiu J, Hsieh MH, Meisel L, Oliveira IC, Shin M, Coruzzi G. Glutamate-receptor genes in plants. Nature. 1998;**396**:125-126

[57] Beemster GT, Baskin TI. Analysis of cell division and elongation underlying the developmental acceleration of root growth in *Arabidopsis thaliana*. Plant Physiology. 1998;**116**:1515-1526

[58] Dolan L, Janmaat K, Willemsen V, Linstead P, Poethig S, Roberts K, Scheres B. Cellular organisation of the *Arabidopsis thaliana* root. Development. 1993;**119**:71-84

[59] Gonzalez-Garcia MP, Vilarrasa-Blasi J, Zhiponova M, Divol F, Mora-Garcia S, Russinova E, Cano-Delgado AI. Brassinosteroids control meristem size by promoting cell cycle progression in Arabidopsis roots. Development. 2011;**138**:849-859

[60] Aida M, Beis D, Heidstra R, Willemsen V, Blilou I, Galinha C, Nussaume L, Noh YS, Amasino R, Scheres B. The PLETHORA genes mediate patterning of the Arabidopsis root stem cell niche. Cell. 2004;**119**:109-120

[61] Wysocka-Diller JW, Helariutta Y, Fukaki H, Malamy JE, Benfey PN. Molecular analysis of SCARECROW function reveals a radial patterning mechanism common to root and shoot. Development. 2000;**127**:595-603

[62] Moore R. A morphometric analysis of the redistribution of organelles in columella cells in primary roots of normal seedlings and agravitropic mutants of *Hordeum vulgare*. Journal of Experimental Botany. 1985;**36**:1275-1286

[63] Stahl Y, Wink RH, Ingram GC, Simon R. A signaling module controlling the stem cell niche in Arabidopsis root meristems. Current Biology. 2009;**19**:909-914

[64] Blilou I, Xu J, Wildwater M, Willemsen V, Paponov I, Friml J, Heidstra R, Aida M, Palme K, Scheres B. The PIN auxin efflux facilitator network controls growth and patterning in Arabidopsis roots. Nature. 2005;**433**:39-44

[65] Sabatini S, Beis D, Wolkenfelt H, Murfett J, Guilfoyle T, Malamy J, Benfey P, Leyser O, Bechtold N, Weisbeek P, Scheres B. An auxin-dependent distal organizer of pattern and polarity in the Arabidopsis root. Cell. 1999;**99**:463-472

[66] Swanson GT, Sakai R. Ligands for ionotropic glutamate receptors. Progress in Molecular and Subcellular Biology. 2009;**46**:123-157

[67] Demidchik V, Essah PA, Tester M. Glutamate activates cation currents in the plasma membrane of Arabidopsis root cells. Planta. 2004;**219**:167-175

[68] Weisenberg RC. Microtubule formation in vitro in solutions containing low calcium concentrations. Science. 1972;**177**:1104-1105

[69] Schapansky J, Morissette M, Odero G, Albensi B, Glazner G. Neuregulin beta1 enhances peak glutamate-induced intracellular calcium levels through endoplasmic reticulum calcium release in cultured hippocampal neurons. Canadian Journal of Physiology and Pharmacology. 2009;**87**:883-891

[70] Trewavas AJ, Malho R. Ca^{2+} signalling in plant cells: The big network! Current Opinion in Plant Biology. 1998;**1**:428-433

[71] Xu J, Brearley CA, Lin WH, Wang Y, Ye R, Mueller-Roeber B, Xu ZH, Xue HW. A role of Arabidopsis inositol polyphosphate kinase, AtIPK2alpha, in pollen germination and root growth. Plant Physiology. 2005;**137**:94-103

[72] Lee JS, Mulkey TJ, Evans ML. Reversible loss of gravitropic sensitivity in maize roots after tip application of calcium chelators. Science. 1983;**220**:1375-1376

[73] Roy SJ, Gilliham M, Berger B, Essah PA, Cheffings C, Miller AJ, Davenport RJ, Liu LH, Skynner MJ, Davies JM, Richardson P, Leigh RA, Tester M. Investigating glutamate receptor-like gene co-expression in *Arabidopsis thaliana*. Plant, Cell & Environment. 2008;**31**:861-871

[74] Dela Fuente RK, Leopold AC. A role for calcium in auxin transport. Plant Physiology. 1973;**51**:845-847

[75] Casimiro I, Marchant A, Bhalerao RP, Beeckman T, Dhooge S, Swarup R, Graham N, Inze D, Sandberg G, Casero PJ, Bennett M. Auxin transport promotes Arabidopsis lateral root initiation. Plant Cell. 2001;**13**:843-852

[76] Muday GK, Haworth P. Tomato root growth, gravitropism, and lateral development: Correlation with auxin transport. Plant Physiology and Biochemistry. 1994;**32**:193-203

[77] Reed RC, Brady SR, Muday GK. Inhibition of auxin movement from the shoot into the root inhibits lateral root development in Arabidopsis. Plant Physiology. 1998;**118**:1369-1378

Chapter 5

GABA and Glutamate: Their Transmitter Role in the CNS and Pancreatic Islets

Christiane S. Hampe, Hiroshi Mitoma and Mario Manto

Additional information is available at the end of the chapter

http://dx.doi.org/10.5772/intechopen.70958

Abstract

Glutamate and gamma-aminobutyric acid (GABA) are the major neurotransmitters in the mammalian brain. Inhibitory GABA and excitatory glutamate work together to control many processes, including the brain's overall level of excitation. The contributions of GABA and glutamate in extra-neuronal signaling are by far less widely recognized. In this chapter, we first discuss the role of both neurotransmitters during development, emphasizing the importance of the shift from excitatory to inhibitory GABAergic neurotransmission. The second part summarizes the biosynthesis and role of GABA and glutamate in neurotransmission in the mature brain, and major neurological disorders associated with glutamate and GABA receptors and GABA release mechanisms. The final part focuses on extra-neuronal glutamatergic and GABAergic signaling in pancreatic islets of Langerhans, and possible associations with type 1 diabetes mellitus.

Keywords: glutamate, GABA, CNS, pancreatic islets, neurological disorders autoimmune diabetes

1. Introduction

Glutamate and gamma-aminobutyric acid (GABA) are the major neurotransmitters in the brain. Inhibitory GABA and excitatory glutamate work together to control many processes, including the brain's overall level of excitation. A balanced interaction is required to maintain the physiological homeostasis, while prolonged imbalance can lead to disease. Glutamatergic/GABAergic imbalance can be found in autism spectrum disorders and anxiety disorders with elevated glutamatergic neurotransmission, while high levels of GABA produce more relaxation and even sedation. Neurotransmitter levels can be affected by external factors, for example, alcohol. Alcohol potentiates the sedentary effects of GABA, while inhibiting the excitatory aspects of glutamate, resulting in an overall increase in GABA/glutamate ratio. This leads to sensations of relaxation and in later stages to loss of control with slurred speech, unsteady gait and loss of social anxiety. The GABA/glutamate balance can also be affected by autoimmunity and genetic disorders. The contributions of GABA and glutamate in extra-neuronal signaling are by far less recognized. We will discuss extra-neuronal GABAergic and glutamatergic signaling and its relevance in insulin secretion from the pancreatic islets of Langerhans.

2. Glutamate and GABA during development

Both glutamatergic and GABAergic neurons are highly diversified in the central nervous system (CNS). More than half a century after the discovery of the effects of GABA, it is now established that in mature neurons, neuronal excitability is characterized by a balance between glutamatergic excitatory input and GABAergic inhibitory transmission. This balance is reached during development. However, the functions of GABAergic signaling are not restricted to a pure inhibitory mechanism at the synaptic level. This is a too simplistic view. For instance, GABA influences patterns and oscillations that are very relevant from the behavioral point of view [1]. GABA and glutamate expression are already widespread in the embryonic stage, and glutamate receptors are expressed in neurons even before glutamatergic synaptogenesis [1]. While glutamate receptor activities tune the developing GABAergic synapse [2], GABA is now considered the main excitatory transmitter during early development, acting not only at a synaptic and network level, but also on cell cycle and migration [1]. This excitatory function of GABA is caused by elevated neuronal intracellular chloride concentration at the early stages of development. The efflux of chloride mediated by GABA in immature neurons is excitatory, triggering sodium spikes and activating voltage-gated Ca^{2+} channels [1]. With time, a progressive reduction of chloride efflux occurs. This explains the shift from a depolarizing to a hyperpolarizing effect. Obata and colleagues were the first to suggest this developmentally regulated shift at the level of the spinal cord [3]. Neuronal chloride homeostasis is regulated by channels, exchangers and co-transporters. The developmental changes of sodium-potassium-chloride cotransporter 1 (NKCC1) (ensuring chloride uptake; higher expression in immature neurons) and potassium-chloride transporter 2 (KCC2) (principal chloride extruder; higher expression in mature neurons) are the masterpieces for the changes in chloride efflux associated with maturation. The developmental shift from local to large-scale network activity occurs in parallel with a gradual shift from electrical to chemical synaptic transmission [4].

It is noteworthy that in immature neurons activation of $GABA_A$ receptors leads to an increase in the intra-cellular concentration of Ca^{2+}, as a consequence of the stimulation of voltage-gated Ca^{2+} channels, which exerts trophic effects on neuritic growth, migration and synaptogenesis. Blocking the $GABA_A$ receptor reduces the cytoplasmic concentrations of Ca^{2+} [5]. In addition, the activation of $GABA_B$ receptors depresses the $GABA_A$ receptor-mediated Ca^{2+} increase and therefore the $GABA_B$ pathway is likely supervising the entry of Ca^{2+} [6]. In granule cells of the cerebellum, the changes in the concentrations of Ca^{2+} outlast the exposure to GABA by several minutes [7]. The $GABA_A$-activated Ca^{2+} influx regulates the expression of the chloride extruder KCC2 [8]. One example of the relevance of this physiological shift in the chloride gradient occurs during delivery when the maternal hormone oxytocin triggers labor [9].

The electrical activity of neurons is a guide for the genesis of neuronal connections. Indeed, neuronal activity exerts a key role in the development of inhibitory GABAergic synapses, interacting closely with genetic programs. Blocking neuronal activity in developing neurons decreases the density of inhibitory synapses, confirming an activity-dependent development [10, 11]. The expression of GABAergic plasticity is related to modifications in the quantity of neurotransmitter in individual vesicles. Migrating neurons express, already at an early stage, both GABA and glutamate receptors [1], but GABA receptors are likely to be established first [12]. Interestingly, tangentially migrating interneurons express AMPA but not GABA or NMDA receptors. Therefore, a modulation/targeting of neurons via selective activation of receptors can be achieved [13]. This has implications for understanding and treatment of migrating disorders affecting the nervous system.

The building of brain networks is a highly complex task which requires organized sequential events, both spatially and from a timing standpoint. While an overdrive of GABAergic signaling slows the development, the overactivity of glutamatergic signaling causes excitotoxicity [1]. GABA receptors are the first to be active, even when synapses are still non-operant. This creates a shunting effect preventing excitotoxicity, since the Na^+ and Ca^{2+} spikes triggered by GABA require only a 30–40 mV driving force. Such a shunt is part of the synergistic interactions between GABA and glutamate. Thanks to these interactions, the neuronal networks in development generate primitive patterns of discharges, observed *in vivo* and in cultured networks, such as the giant depolarizing potentials (GDPs) which allow the building of functional units [1]. GDPs resemble interictal-like epileptiform discharges and provide synchronous Ca^{2+} oscillations also contributing to the development of networks. GDPs rely on the release of GABA, glutamate, and glycine at the onset of synaptogenesis [14]. The synchronized activity is one of the factors controlling the phenomenon of maturation [11]. Synchronization is also achieved, thanks to gap junctions, intrinsic voltage-dependent conductance [15], and non-vesicular paracrine release of neurotransmitters [16].

The capacity of developing nervous system to generate spontaneous activity in absence of external stimulation is a remarkable feature that has been observed in particular in the retina, the cerebral cortex, the hippocampus, the cerebellum, the hindbrain, and the spinal cord [14]. Recent works highlight that network bursts are driven by AMPA pathways in terms of coordination, whereas the shaping of the dynamics of spiking activities is regulated by NMDA- and GABA-associated currents [17].

3. Glutamate and GABA in the mature mammalian brain

3.1. Biosynthesis of glutamate and GABA: the glutamate/GABA-glutamine cycle

Glutamate and GABA do not cross the blood-brain barrier and must therefore be synthesized within the CNS. As neurons lack the enzyme pyruvate carboxylase and therefore cannot synthesize glutamate through the TCA cycle [18], they rely on astrocytes for the generation of glutamate. Astrocytes generate glutamate via *de novo* synthesis or by "recycling" glutamine from GABA and glutamate after reuptake. However, *de novo* synthesis makes up only ~15% of astrocytic glutamate [19]. In this reaction, pyruvate is generated from glucose during glycolysis and enters the TCA after conversion to Acetyl CoA. The TCA product α-ketoglutarate can be converted to glutamate, which is converted to glutamine by glutamine synthetase, an enzyme that is predominately, if not exclusively, located in astrocytes [20]. Glutamine exits astrocytes via the bidirectional N system transporters, SNAT3 and SNAT5 [21], and enter neurons via the unidirectional system A transporters, SNAT1, SNAT2 [21], and SNAT7 [22]. There glutamine is converted back to glutamate by phosphate-activated glutaminase, an enzyme which is expressed preferentially in neurons [23]. GABAergic neurons require an additional step to convert glutamate to GABA through decarboxylation. After release from the neurons, GABA and glutamate reenter the astrocytes to be "recycled" to glutamine. A small portion of glutamate is oxidatively metabolized, thus making *de novo* synthesis of glutamate necessary to maintain adequate glutamate levels [24]. The continuous recycling of glutamate, GABA and glutamine between neurons and astrocytes is known as the glutamate/GABA-glutamine cycle [25] (**Figure 1**).

3.2. Glutamatergic neurotransmission

In glutamatergic neurons, glutamate is packaged into synaptic vesicles (SVs) by vesicular glutamate transporters (VGLUT1–3) [26]. The loaded SVs then dock near the release site, where they are primed into a state of competence for Ca^{2+}-triggered fusion-pore opening. Once glutamate has been released, SVs can either fully collapse into the synaptic membrane, or close rapidly and undock ("kiss-and-run") [27].

Released glutamate is recognized by glutamate receptors (GluRs). Binding of glutamate changes the receptor's conformation and allows influx of extracellular Na^+ and other cations, and an efflux of intracellular K^+ ions. GluRs fall into two major categories: ionotropic and metabotropic [28]. Ionotropic GluRs are tetrameric ligand-gated cation channels that induce depolarization of the postsynaptic membrane. The three types of ionotropic GluRs are named

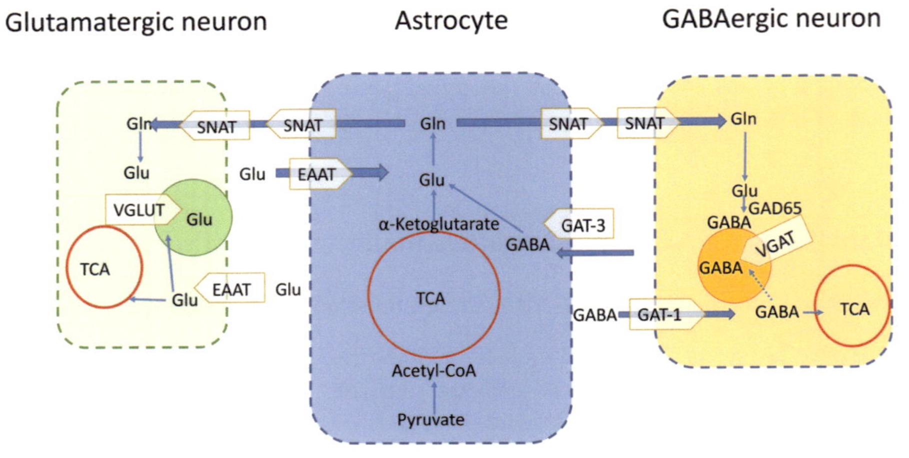

Figure 1. Overview of the glutamate/GABA-glutamine cycle. For details see text.

after ligands that selectively bind to one receptor only: N-methyl-D-aspartate (NMDA), alpha-amino-3-hydroxy-5-methyl-4-isoxazolepropionic acid (AMPA), and Kainate, however all three are bound by glutamate [28]. NMDA receptors (NMDA-Rs) activate slower than AMPA and Kainate receptors. This delayed reaction is caused by the blockage of the cation pore of NMDA-Rs by external Mg^{2+} at resting membrane potential, which is removed upon depolarization of the neurons [29, 30]. Thus, non-NMDA-Rs activation is necessary to depolarize the neurons allowing NMDA-Rs activation. NMDA-Rs also close slower than non-NMDA-Rs, and therefore determine the duration of the synaptic current.

NMDA-Rs also allow influx of Ca^{2+} and have thereby a regulatory role in synaptic plasticity by connecting synaptic activity with Ca^{2+}-mediated biochemical signaling [31]. Depending on the nature of the neuron's depolarization, NMDA-Rs can both strengthen synapses, through long-term potentiation (LTP) [32, 33], and weaken synapses, through long-term depression (LTD) [34]. For LTP, repetitive and strong depolarization of the neurons allows significant influx of Ca^{2+} into the cytoplasm and activation of protein kinases, including the calcium/calmodulin-dependent protein kinase II (CaMKII), which (a) phosphorylate and activate AMPA-Rs and (b) trigger the insertion of additional AMPA-Rs into the postsynaptic membrane [35]. This increases the postsynaptic neuron's responsiveness to glutamate leading to LTP. By strengthening the neighboring connections of similar activity patterns, the NMDA-R enforces the Hebbian postulate that 'cells that fire together, wire together' [36]. For LTD, weak depolarization by low frequency stimulation still activates NMDA-Rs, but promotes only a modest prolonged increase in Ca^{2+} levels. Protein phosphatases (protein phosphatase 1 and protein phosphatase calcineurin) have a much higher affinity for calcium/calmodulin compared to CaMKII and are activated at lower Ca^{2+} levels. Thus, under the above conditions protein phosphatases are activated [37], dephosphorylate AMPA-Rs, and induce the removal of AMPA-Rs from the postsynaptic membrane [38], thereby reducing the postsynaptic responsiveness to glutamate and leading to LTD.

Metabotropic glutamate receptors (mGluRs) [39] are overall slower acting than iGluRs. In difference to iGluRs, mGluRs are not ion channels, but belong to a group of G-protein-coupled receptors. The associated G-protein consists of three subunits (α, β, and γ), of which the α-subunit is associated with GDP. Glutamate binding to the receptor induces a conformational change that allows the replacement of GDP with GTP and consequent dissociation of the three G-protein subunits. While the $G_{\beta/\gamma}$-complex activates K^+ and Na^+ channels, the α-subunit interacts with different enzymes [40]. Excitatory G_α-subunits ($G_{\alpha q}$ or $G_{\alpha 11}$) bind and activate phospholipase C-β (PLC-β), initiating a signaling cascade leading to the activation of protein kinase C (PKC) and the release of Ca^{2+} from the ER. Another excitatory G_α-subunit ($G_{\alpha s}$) activates the membrane-associated adenylyl cyclase, which catalyzes the conversion of ATP to cAMP, leading to activation of protein kinase A (PKA). Inhibiting G_α-subunits ($G_{\alpha i}$ or $G_{\alpha o}$) prevent activation of adenylyl cyclase and the activation of PKA [41]. The three mGluRs groups (I–III) differ in their alpha subunits. Generally, Group I mGluRs carry activating $G_{\alpha s}$ or $G_{\alpha 11}$ subunits, are localized postsynaptically, and lead to cell depolarization and increased neuronal excitability. Groups II and III mGluRs carry inhibitory $G_{\alpha i}$ or $G_{\alpha o}$ subunits and are often localized on presynaptic terminals or preterminal axons, where they inhibit neurotransmitter release [42].

Released glutamate must be rapidly removed to avoid continuous stimulation and excitotoxicity [43, 44] (see also glutamate-induced excitotoxicity). Glutamate uptake is mediated via brain excitatory amino acid transporters (EAATs) on both pre- and postsynaptic neurons and on surrounding astrocytes [45]. Five subtypes of EAATs (EAAT1–5) have been cloned so far. A smaller portion of extracellular glutamate is reabsorbed by presynaptic or postsynaptic neurons.

Another mechanism involved in the extracellular glutamate regulation is the cystine/glutamate exchange transporter xc(−). In contrast to the EAATs, xc(−) is involved in elevating extracellular glutamate concentrations. Here intracellular glutamate is exchanged for extracellular cystine. The stimulation of xc(−) modulates glutamate release from the presynaptic neurons [46]. xc(−) regulates glutamate homeostasis through the involvement of the presynaptic mGluR2/3. Moreover, a decrease of xc(−) expression can lead to a reduction in extrasynaptic glutamate level. This effect may cause a loss of glutamatergic tone on presynaptic mGluR2/3, which can lead to a marked increase in glutamate release from presynaptic glutamatergic neurons [47].

3.3. GABAergic neurotransmission

For the synthesis of GABA, glutamate is decarboxylated to GABA by glutamate decarboxylase (GAD). GAD is expressed as two isoforms (GAD67 and GAD65) and can be found only in GABAergic neurons and in certain peripheral tissues, most prominently in the pancreatic islets [48]. GABA can also be taken up by presynaptic neurons after its release into the synapsis. However, this recycled GABA is mainly metabolized to generate ATP through the GABA shunt pathway [49], while newly synthesized GABA is preferentially taken up into SVs [49]. Transport of newly synthesized GABA into SVs is tightly linked to its synthesis, as GAD65 and the GABA transporter VGAT form a protein complex with chaperone protein HSC70, the vesicular cysteine string protein (CSP), and CaMKII [49]. In the absence of GAD65 from this complex, the active site of VGAT may be available to cytosolic GABA, and vesicular transport of GABA can be restored to a certain extent [49]. GAD65 has also a crucial role in the trafficking of GABAergic vesicles to presynaptic clusters [50]. Palmitoylation of cysteine residues located at the N-terminus of GAD65 is required for the transport of GAD65 to synaptic terminals [51], and decreased palmitoylation impairs GABAergic neurotransmission, as observed in Huntington's disease [52]. Similar to glutamate, GABA is released in a Ca^{2+}-dependent manner upon depolarization of the presynaptic membrane.

GABA receptors present as ionotropic $GABA_A$ receptors that cause rapid inhibitory postsynaptic potentials, and metabotropic $GABA_B$ receptors that cause slow inhibitory postsynaptic potentials [53]. $GABA_A$ receptors are multi-subunit proteins [54] and consist of three major subunits (α, β, and γ). A total of five subunits are arranged around the central ion pore. The major receptor isoform consists of two α_1, two β_2, and one γ_2 subunits. GABA binding to $GABA_A$ receptors on the postsynaptic neuron induces rapid and transient opening of $GABA_A$ receptor Cl^- channels [55]. The subsequent influx of anions hyperpolarizes the membrane (phasic inhibition). GABA overspill can activate extrasynaptical $GABA_A$ receptors, inducing a more prolonged opening of the ion channel (tonic inhibition) [56].

Metabotropic G-protein coupled $GABA_B$ receptors are mostly located extrasynaptically and can be found both pre- and the postsynaptical. These heterodimers consist of $GABA_{B1}$ and $GABA_{B2}$ subunits. The $GABA_{B1}$ subunit can be bound by GABA, while $GABA_{B2}$ is coupled to the G-protein. Activation of $GABA_B$ receptors induces the dissociation of the subunits of the coupled G-protein. The $G_{\beta/\gamma}$-subunit complex activates inwardly rectifying K^+ channels [57] and inhibits voltage-activated Ca^{2+} channels [58], resulting in hyperpolarization of the neuron and inhibition of neurotransmission [59]. The $G_{\alpha i}$-subunit inhibits activation of adenylyl cyclase as described above for mGluR. Activation of presynaptical $GABA_B$ receptors impedes opening of voltage-activated Ca^{2+} channels and thereby reduces neurotransmitter release. Thus GABA can inhibit its own release through a negative feedback loop via $GABA_B$ receptors present on GABAergic axons [60]. Activation of postsynaptical $GABA_B$ receptors reduces depolarization of the plasma membrane and thereby modulates excitatory signals.

The reuptake of GABA is mediated by GABA transporter protein present in presynaptic nerve terminals (GAT-1) and surrounding glial cells (GAT-3) [61].

3.4. Neurological diseases associated with glutamate and GABA receptors and GABA release mechanisms

3.4.1. *Limbic encephalitis*

The relation between anti-GluR antibodies (Abs) with limbic encephalitis has been investigated during the last two decades [62, 63]. Several autoantibodies against extracellular epitopes of GluR involved in synaptic transmission and plasticity, such as AMPA-Rs [64] and NMDA-Rs [65] are described. The affected patients develop complex neuropsychiatric symptoms, such as memory deficits, cognition impairment, psychosis, seizures, abnormal movements, or coma. These disorders affect mainly young women, though cases of men and children have been reported [62]. Some of these patients present with malignant tumors and the syndrome can be qualified as paraneoplastic [62], characterized by association of anti-NMDA-RAb in ovarian teratoma and anti-AMPA-RAb in lung small cell carcinoma. Paraneoplastic limbic encephalitis can be fatal, but is curable if treated at an early stage by surgical removal of the tumor and a combination of immunotherapeutic agents [62]. Mechanistically, autoantibodies directed against AMPA-Rs and NMDA-Rs decrease the numbers of the cell-surface receptors [63] and anti-AMPA-RAb may act as agonists and increase cell excitability [66].

3.4.2. *Immune-mediated cerebellar ataxias*

Compared with autoimmune encephalitis affecting the limbic system, autoantibodies to GluRs, such as anti-mGluR1 Ab and anti-glutamate receptor delta2 (GluRδ2) Ab, are less frequently associated with immune-mediated cerebellar ataxias (IMCAs). Anti-mGluR1Ab was reported in two patients with malignant lymphoma and one patient with prostate adenocarcinoma [67, 68]. Anti-mGluR1Ab impairs the induction of LTD, which causes ataxia in mice [67]. Interestingly, IMCAs associated with anti-GluRδ2Ab are always preceded or accompanied by either infection or vaccination [58]. Polyclonal Abs toward the putative ligand-binding site of GluRδ2 are known to cause AMPA-R endocytosis and attenuate their synaptic transmission, resulting in the development of ataxia in mice [69].

3.4.3. *Autosomal recessive cerebellar degeneration*

Autosomal recessive CAs (ARCAs) are affected by several gene mutations. One of these involves mutations in the GRM1 gene, which encodes mGluR1, known to play an important role in cerebellar differentiation [70]. Accordingly, the clinical features of this familial form of CAs appear already during childhood. The child shows global developmental delay, intellectual defects, severe CAs, and pyramidal signs. Brain imaging often shows progressive generalized cerebellar atrophy. Mutations affect a gene region critical for alternative splicing and the formation of the receptor structure.

3.4.4. *Glutamate-induced excitotoxicity*

Deficits and mutations in GluR can also affect the level of extracellular glutamate with detrimental outcomes for neurotransmission and neuronal health. The level of extracellular glutamate is determined by three factors: (1) vesicular-released glutamate at the synapses, (2) non-vesicular-released glutamate from the system xc(−) (see above) [71], and (3) glutamate uptake by EAATs on astrocytes [72]. When glutamate release exceeds glutamate uptake, the excess glutamate activates a large number of postsynaptic NMDA-Rs, resulting in the induction of excitotoxic neuronal death by allowing excessive Ca^{2+} influx through the receptor-operated cation channels [73]. Excessive activation of NMDA-Rs and the associated Ca^{2+} influx result in stimulation of calpain I and nNOS [73]. This causes DNA damage and formation of ONOO— due to excess NO (nitrosative stress) and other free radicals. The combination of these two changes ultimately leads to mitochondrial dysfunction and cell death [73]. Recent studies reported the presence of high glutamate levels in the extracellular space in chronic degenerative diseases, such as amyotrophic lateral sclerosis, Alzheimer's disease, and Huntington's disease [74]. Taken together, glutamate-induced excitotoxicity may be a common process for neuronal death throughout the CNS and accelerates the original pathological changes.

3.4.5. *Neurological diseases associated with deficits in GABA receptors*

Anti-$GABA_B$ receptor Ab is associated with limbic encephalitis [75], which manifests clinically similar to anti-GluRAb-mediated limbic encephalitis. Some patients also develop CAs. About 50% of the patients have neoplastic diseases, especially small cell lung carcinoma [75]. Clinical studies indicate that surgical removal of the lung tumor and subsequent immunotherapy can be effective in the relief of the above neurological disorders, especially in the early stages of disease.

3.4.6. *Association of GAD65 dysfunction with neurological disorders*

Anti-GAD65Abs are associated with stiff-person syndrome (SPS) and CAs [76]. Titers of anti-GAD65Ab are high (>1000 U/ml) in both conditions. SPS is characterized clinically by progressive rigidity and painful-muscle spasms in the axial and limb muscles. Electromyography (EMG) shows simultaneous activities of the agonist and antagonistic muscles. Anti-GAD65Ab-associated

CAs affect mostly women in their 50–60s and exhibit subacute or chronic CAs, which are sometimes associated with SPS or epilepsy [76]. Furthermore, the majority of patients also suffer from type 1 diabetes mellitus (T1D) [76].

Based on the intracellular location of GAD65 (on the cytoplasmic side of SVs), the pathogenic role of anti-GAD65Ab in CA and SPS has been questioned. However, recent studies have shed new light on this issue. First, the pathogenic actions of anti-GAD65Ab have been clarified both in *in vitro* and *in vivo* preparations [77–82], for example, the Cerebrospinal fluid (CSF) of patients with SPS inhibited GABA synthesis [83]. Furthermore, SPS-like symptoms were reproduced in experimental rats and mice injected intrathecally or intraventricularly [84] or intracerebellarly [80] with IgGs obtained from the CSF of CA and SPS patients. Specifically, IgGs obtained from the CSF of patients with anti-GAD65Ab-associated CA depressed GABA release in cerebellar brain slices [77, 78, 82, 85], and their intracerebellar injection interfered with cerebellar control of the motor cortex and resulted in ataxic gait in rats [79]. These actions were reproduced by human anti-GAD65 monoclonal Ab b78, which binds to an epitope similar to that recognized in SPS patients positive for anti-GAD65Ab [80–82].

Second, studies in animals have shown internalization of antibodies by cerebellar neurons [81, 86], demonstrating that anti-GAD65Ab can access their intracellular target. Together, these results indicate the possibility that anti-GAD65Ab may damage sufficient numbers of GABAergic neurons to result in the appearance of frank neurological symptoms [87].

The pathological effects of anti-GAD65Ab depend on epitope specificity. Specifically, the pathologic effects of anti-GAD65Abs on GABA synthesis and release were specific to anti-GAD65Ab b78—representing SPS- and CA-associated anti-GAD65Ab—and could not be reproduced by monoclonal anti-GAD65Ab b96.11, representing an epitope specificity associated with type 1 diabetes mellitus [80–82]. This epitope dependence might explain the differences in neurological phenotypes. Administration of CSF obtained from patients with SPS or CAs reproduced the clinical features of the corresponding disease in mice [80]. Thus anti-GAD65Ab in SPS that inhibit GABA synthesis, would attenuate inhibitory Purkinje cell-mediated depression of the spino-cerebellar loop, resulting in increased muscle tone, whereas anti-GAD65Ab in CAs depress GABA release, resulting in disruption of Purkinje cell-mediated modulation of the cerebro-cerebellar loop to elicit disorganized movements [87]. An alternative explanation of the phenotypic differences is the involvement of other autoimmune-mediated mechanisms.

In anti-GAD65Ab-associated CAs, anti-GAD65Ab impairs the association of GAD65 with the cytosolic side of SVs resulting in a decrease in vesicular GABA contents with low release probability [82]. Under normal conditions, the released GABA spills over to the neighboring excitatory synaptic terminals and inhibits presynaptic glutamate release through GABA receptors. However, this GABA-induced inhibition of glutamate release is disturbed in patients with CAs [77]. Taken together, anti-GAD65Ab elicit marked imbalance in neurotransmitters; including a decrease in GABA and an increase in glutamate. The imbalance between GABA and glutamate is accelerated following the involvement of microglia and astrocytes [87]. Microglia activated by excessive glutamate levels can secrete various cytokines, which facilitate glutamate release presumably through xc(−) on microglia, and suppress the uptake of glutamate through EAATs on astrocytes [71, 88, 89]. Thus, the neuroinflammation-induced chain reactions accelerate the imbalance, leading to profound excitotoxicity. In agreement with this notion, the cerebellar neurons are completely lost in patients with advanced stage CAs [90].

In conclusion, deficits in glutamate- and GABA-mediated synaptic mechanisms, upset the glutamate/GABA ratio. Notably, the level of glutamate is relatively high compared with that of GABA, caused by various etiologies, including glutamate release by damage-induced depolarization, exaggerated glutamate release through xc(−), and attenuated uptake of glutamate through EAATs, or a decrease in GABA release with subsequent increase in glutamate release. The imbalance between glutamate and GABA can trigger excitotoxicity, one of several neuron death mechanisms.

4. GABA/glutamate signaling pathways in pancreatic islets and implications in type 1 diabetes mellitus

While GABA and glutamate are best characterized for their role as neurotransmitter, they are also involved in extra-neuronal signaling. As a major building block in proteins synthesis, intracellular glutamate is abundantly present in the body. In contrast, GABA is present only in restricted non-neuronal tissues, including the pancreas [91]. Pancreatic islets are clusters of endocrine cells located in the exocrine pancreas and regulate blood glucose homeostasis. An islet typically contains insulin-releasing beta cells, glucagon-secreting alpha cells, somatostatin-containing delta cells, and pancreatic polypeptide-producing (PP) cells. The metabolic actions of insulin and glucagon are reviewed in great detail elsewhere [92]. Briefly, insulin is released at elevated blood glucose levels and acts as an anabolic hormone, causing cellular glucose uptake primarily in skeletal muscles, the liver, and fat tissue. Here glucose is converted to storable energy substrates including glycogen and triglycerides, respectively. At low blood glucose levels, glucagon is secreted from pancreatic alpha cells. Glucagon causes the liver to convert stored glycogen to glucose and induces lipolysis in fat tissue. Many regulatory mechanisms are in place to control the secretion of insulin and glucagon to maintain stable blood glucose levels. Within the islet, extracellular insulin inhibits glucagon secretion from alpha cells, while glucagon enhances both insulin and somatostatin secretion [93]. In recent years, GABA and glutamate have gained interest for their respective roles in the regulation of secretion of insulin and glucagon.

In the following sections, we will review GABAergic and glutamatergic signaling in the islets of Langerhans and possible implications for type 1 diabetes mellitus.

4.1. Glutamate and GABA in pancreatic islets

Both glutamate and GABA are synthesized from glucose taken up by beta cells. The majority of glucose is metabolized to produce energy, however a portion is converted to glutamate. The initial step is catalyzed by pyruvate carboxylase present in the beta cells [94]. Thus, in contrast to GABAergic neurons, beta cells can synthesize glutamate on their own. In the alpha cells, glutamate is loaded into glucagon-containing secretory granules via VGLUT1 and VGLUT2

[95]. Within the beta cells, glutamate is decarboxylated by GAD to yield GABA. GABA is packaged by the GABA transporter VGAT into small synaptic-like microvesicles (SLMVs) [96]. A smaller fraction of GABA is present in insulin-containing large dense core vesicles (LDCVs) [97, 98]. These vesicles also express VGAT, suggesting similar packaging mechanisms as for SLMVs [98]. GABA is present predominantly, if not exclusively, in the beta cells [96, 99, 100], and GABA and GAD expression levels in beta cells are similar to those in GABAergic neurons [97].

Both isoforms of GAD have been identified in pancreatic beta cells, GAD65 being the predominant isoform in rat and human beta cells, while mice beta cells only express GAD67 [48]. In human and rat beta cells GAD65 co-localizes with GABA at the SLMVs [101], while in murine pancreatic islets, GAD67 is firmly membrane anchored and efficiently transits to presynaptic clusters [102]. It remains unclear whether GAD is involved in SLMVs transport to the plasma membrane, in analogy to GABAergic neurons (see also Section 3.3).

As outlined above, GABA is present in both SLMVs and insulin-containing LDCVs. The basal release of GABA from beta cells is relatively constant [101, 103], but can be modulated depending on the metabolic state of the cell [104]. The mechanisms involved in GABA release were first investigated in beta cell lines, where GABA secretion was shown to be dependent on the presence of extracellular Ca^{2+} [105], suggesting that GABA is released in response to an increase in cytosolic Ca^{2+} levels. A detection system for GABA release involving overexpressed $GABA_A$ receptors in dispersed rat islets allowed the sensitive detection of GABA release as fluctuations in current in whole-cell patch-clamped beta cells [106]. These studies confirmed that GABA release is dependent on the entry of extracellular Ca^{2+} through voltage-gated channels and not by membrane depolarization itself. The study further indicated that the observed GABA release originated predominantly from SLMVs rather than LDCVs.

Both beta and alpha cells express $GABA_A$ and $GABA_B$ receptors [103]. Through the expression of GABA receptors on beta cells, GABA regulates its own secretion (autocrine regulation). $GABA_A$ receptor activation induces further GABA release (autocrine positive feedback loop) [97, 107]. However, GABA-mediated regulation of GABA release depends on the extracellular glucose concentration. At high glucose concentrations, GABA hyperpolarizes the membrane of isolated beta cells and beta cell lines [108]. This inhibitory effects appears be mediated via $GABA_B$ receptors [106, 109].

Presence of GABA receptors on adjacent alpha cells enables a paracrine regulation of these cells [110]. Activation of $GABA_A$ receptors on alpha cells leads to hyperpolarization and suppression of glucagon and glutamate secretion [103, 111]. As glucagon and glutamate trigger insulin release from beta cells, GABAergic inhibition of glucagon and glutamate secretion indirectly downregulates insulin release from beta cells as a negative feedback regulation (**Figure 2**). Extracellular GABA is taken up by the plasma membrane GABA transporter GAT3 expressed on both alpha and beta cells [98].

At low concentrations of glucose, alpha cells show high action potentials [103, 112], mediated by voltage-gated Na^+ and Ca^{2+} channels [113]. This triggers the release of glucagon and glutamate. At high glucose concentrations, release of glucagon and glutamate is inhibited,

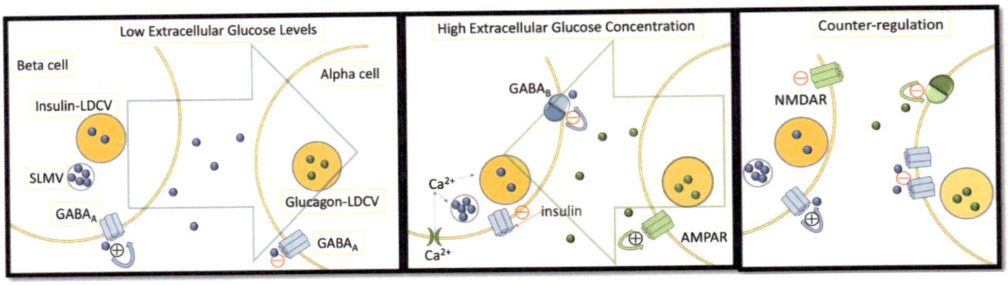

Figure 2. Schematic outline of presumed GABAergic and glutamatergic signaling in pancreatic islets. At low glucose concentrations, beta cells release GABA in a glucose-independent manner [97, 108]. This tonic GABA release continuously activates GABA$_A$ receptors on beta cells and alpha cells. GABA$_A$ receptor activation leads to further GABA release from beta cells and suppresses release of glucagon and glutamate from alpha cells, thereby preventing insulin secretion. As extracellular glucose levels rise, the level of intracellular Ca^{2+} increases in beta cells, allowing release of insulin. Secreted insulin inhibits GABA$_A$ receptors on the beta cells, thereby decreasing the autocrine positive feedback release of GABA from beta cells and reducing GABA-mediated inhibition of alpha cells [140]. Moreover, under high glucose concentrations GABA inhibits its own release from beta cells (via GABA$_B$ receptor activation). Reduced extracellular GABA concentrations allow glucagon and glutamate secretion from alpha cells. Glutamate triggers glutamate and glucagon release via activation of AMPA-Rs and glucagon stimulates further insulin release from beta cells. Counter-regulation: eventually, the depolarization of beta cells activates NMDA-Rs present on beta cells, initiating the repolarization of beta cells and limiting insulin release. Reduced insulin levels lift the inhibition of GABA$_A$ receptors on beta cells and allow positive feedback regulation of GABA release. Elevated extracellular GABA levels can now activate GABA$_A$ receptors on alpha cells and inhibit glutamate and glucagon release. Of note, insulin secretion induces GABA$_A$ receptors phosphorylation and translocation to alpha cell plasma membrane [111]. This renders alpha cells more susceptible to GABA-mediated suppression of glucagon secretion, and ultimately limits insulin secretion from beta cells [111, 141].

although the mechanistic details of this regulation remain unclear. Paracrine GABA-mediated regulation (as described above) is suggested by the finding that isolated rat alpha cells no longer show reduced glucagon/glutamate release at elevated glucose concentrations [112], and the observation that in rat islets and purified alpha cells, GABA antagonists suppress glucagon secretion [114]. Insulin and GABA are suggested to serve as paracrine inhibitors of glutamate and glucagon release [101, 103, 115].

Once released, glutamate activates GluRs expressed on both alpha and beta cells. The cell-specific distribution of AMPA-R/Kainate receptors and NMDA-Rs remains debated, and earlier reports suggested that AMPA-Rs are expressed exclusively on alpha cells, while NMDA-Rs were reported to be specifically expressed on beta cells [116]. However, later reports suggest that AMPA-Rs are also expressed on mouse beta cells, and other studies suggest iGluRs expression only on alpha and not on beta cells [117]. mGluRs mGluR8, mGluR5 and mGluR2/3 are expressed by beta cells [109, 118], while mGluR4 protein is expressed on alpha cells [119]. Extracellular glutamate activates AMPA/kainate Rs present on alpha cells and triggers the co-release of glutamate and glucagon (positive feedback regulation) [117, 120, 121]. On the other hand, activation of mGluR inhibits glucagon/glutamate secretion from alpha cells [119] (negative feedback regulation). Few studies reported that activation of AMPA/Kainate-R and/or mGluR on beta cells triggers insulin secretion [118, 120], however subsequent studies could not confirm these results [117]. Still, through glucagon-mediated insulin release from beta cells, co-secreted glutamate indirectly stimulates insulin secretion from beta cells [121]. In addition, glutamate stimulates GABA release from SLMVs in beta cells independently of insulin release,

http://dx.doi.org/10.5772/intechopen.70958

thus serving as a regulatory factor to limit glucagon/glutamate release [106]. As in the GABAergic system, glutamate-mediated regulation of beta cells depends on the extracellular glucose concentration. The high-affinity NMDA-Rs on the beta cell are already saturated at physiological glutamate concentrations in the islet, and are mainly activated through depolarization of beta cells [121]. As islets are depolarized by external glucose, the NMDA-R-mediated repolarization of the beta cells is a negative feedback regulation of glucose-stimulated insulin secretion. Extracellular glutamate is taken up by EAAT1 and 2 expressed on alpha cells [122].

4.2. Proposed GABAergic and glutamatergic signaling in type 1 diabetes mellitus

Type 1 diabetes mellitus (T1D) is an autoimmune disease, characterized by the specific destruction of pancreatic beta cells. Exogenous administration of insulin is necessary to avoid hyperglycemia. Additionally, within 5 years of disease diagnosis, almost all patients with T1D lose their ability to generate an adequate glucagon response to hypoglycemia [123]. This loss has been attributed to the lack of intracellular regulation of beta- to alpha-cell signaling during hypoglycemia [124] and may account for the elevated plasma glucagon levels in diabetes patients, indicating alpha-cell hypersecretion [125, 126]. As observed for neurons, beta cells are sensitive to elevated extracellular glutamate levels and show signs of secretory defects and apoptosis at high glutamate levels [122]. This effect was not prevented by AMPA-R and Kainate-R antagonists and therefore unlikely caused by excitotoxicity. Instead, oxidative stress appears to be the underlying mechanism of glutamate-induced beta-cell death. As outlined in detail in the CNS portion of this chapter, the glutamate/cystine antiporter system xc(−) exchanges intracellular glutamate for extracellular cystine. Excess extracellular glutamate inhibits and/or reverts the activity of the antiporter, thus depleting the cells of cysteine, a building block of the antioxidant glutathione, possibly increasing the cells' vulnerability to oxidative stress [122]. Upregulation of EAAT1 expression on beta cells protects beta cells from glutamate-induced toxicity [122], indicating glutamate signaling as a potential therapeutic target. Notably, many effective antidiabetic drugs such as GLP-1, exenatide, and glitazones also show significant neuroprotective activity against glutamate-induced cytotoxicity in the brain [127, 128]. Moreover, topiramate, an anti-epileptic drug that provides neuroprotection by preventing glutamate toxicity, has antidiabetic and beta-cell cytoprotective effects [129] and long-lasting remission was observed in a T1D patient after treatment with topiramate for generalized seizures [130].

GABA has an overall anti-inflammatory effect on the immune system [131]. $GABA_A$ receptors are expressed by T cells, B cells, and other mononuclear cells, and their activation suppresses lymphocyte proliferation [132, 133]. This GABA-mediated inhibition of T cell responses may provide the mechanism of GABA-associated protection of animal models for development of T1D [134]. GABA also promotes a shift from an inflammatory to an anti-inflammatory cytokine profile *in vivo* and *in vitro* [107]. Another aspect of GABA activity in regard to pancreatic beta cells has been only recently reported. Through activation of $GABA_B$ receptors, GABA significantly increases beta-cell viability [135] and replication [136]. In mouse models, GABA administration prevented and even reversed T1D [107]. One of the involved mechanisms may be GABA-mediated conversion of alpha cells to beta cells [137, 138]. While the details of the mechanisms involved need to be further investigated, these studies open the intriguing potential to use GABA treatment to re-generate beta cells in T1D [139].

It remains unclear what may cause impaired GABAergic and glutamatergic signaling in the pancreatic islets. No mutations of receptors or other elements of the signaling mechanisms have been identified in T1D so far. GAD65Ab are present in the majority of patients with T1D and are regarded as a byproduct of the immune response without significant relevance for the disease progression. However, it is possible that in analogy to their role in neurological disorders, GAD65Ab are taken up by pancreatic beta cells and (a) uncouple the balanced regulation of insulin and glucagon secretion and (b) induce beta cell apoptosis through prolonged exposure to elevated extracellular glutamate levels. Further research is needed to determine whether GAD65Ab have a pathologic role in the development of T1D.

Author details

Christiane S. Hampe[1]*, Hiroshi Mitoma[2] and Mario Manto[3]

*Address all correspondence to: champe@u.washington.edu

1 University of Washington, Seattle, Washington, USA

2 Tokyo Medical University, Tokyo, Japan

3 ULB Erasme, Brussels, Belgium

References

[1] Ben-Ari Y, Gaiarsa JL, Tyzio R, Khazipov R. GABA: A pioneer transmitter that excites immature neurons and generates primitive oscillations. Physiological Reviews. 2007; **87**:1215-1284

[2] Aamodt SM, Shi J, Colonnese MT, Veras W, Constantine-Paton M. Chronic NMDA exposure accelerates development of GABAergic inhibition in the superior colliculus. Journal of Neurophysiology. 2000;**83**:1580-1591

[3] Obata K, Oide M, Tanaka H. Excitatory and inhibitory actions of GABA and glycine on embryonic chick spinal neurons in culture. Brain Research. 1978;**144**:179-184

[4] Luhmann HJ, Sinning A, Yang JW, Reyes-Puerta V, Stüttgen MC, Kirischuk S, Kilb W. Spontaneous neuronal activity in developing neocortical networks: From single cells to large-scale interactions. Front Neural Circuits. 2016;**10**:40

[5] Obrietan K, van den Pol AN. GABA neurotransmission in the hypothalamus: Developmental reversal from Ca^{2+} elevating to depressing. The Journal of Neuroscience. 1995; **15**:5065-5077

[6] Obrietan K, van den Pol AN. GABAB receptor-mediated inhibition of GABAA receptor calcium elevations in developing hypothalamic neurons. Journal of Neurophysiology. 1998;**79**:1360-1370

[7] Connor JA, Tseng HY, Hockberger PE. Depolarization- and transmitter-induced changes in intracellular Ca^{2+} of rat cerebellar granule cells in explant cultures. The Journal of Neuroscience. 1987;**7**:1384-1400

[8] Ganguly K, Schinder AF, Wong ST, Poo M. GABA itself promotes the developmental switch of neuronal GABAergic responses from excitation to inhibition. Cell. 2001;**105**: 521-532

[9] Tyzio R, Cossart R, Khalilov I, Minlebaev M, Hübner CA, Represa A, Ben-Ari Y, Khazipov R. Maternal oxytocin triggers a transient inhibitory switch in GABA signaling in the fetal brain during delivery. Science. 2006;**314**:1788-1792

[10] Hartman KN, Pal SK, Burrone J, Murthy VN. Activity-dependent regulation of inhibitory synaptic transmission in hippocampal neurons. Nature Neuroscience. 2006;**9**:642-649

[11] Spitzer NC. Electrical activity in early neuronal development. Nature. 2006;**444**:707-712

[12] Manent JB, Demarque M, Jorquera I, Pellegrino C, Ben-Ari Y, Aniksztejn L, Represa A. A noncanonical release of GABA and glutamate modulates neuronal migration. The Journal of Neuroscience. 2005;**25**:4755-4765

[13] Manent JB, Jorquera I, Ben-Ari Y, Aniksztejn L, Represa A. Glutamate acting on AMPA but not NMDA receptors modulates the migration of hippocampal interneurons. The Journal of Neuroscience. 2006;**26**:5901-5909

[14] Czarnecki A, Le Corronc H, Rigato C, Le Bras B, Couraud F, Scain AL, Allain AE, Mouffle C, Bullier E, Mangin JM, Branchereau P, Legendre P. Acetylcholine controls GABA-, glutamate-, and glycine-dependent giant depolarizing potentials that govern spontaneous motoneuron activity at the onset of synaptogenesis in the mouse embryonic spinal cord. The Journal of Neuroscience. 2014;**34**:6389-6404

[15] Allene C, Cossart R. Early NMDA receptor-driven waves of activity in the developing neocortex: Physiological or pathological network oscillations? The Journal of Physiology. 2010;**588**:83-91

[16] Scain AL, Le Corronc H, Allain AE, Muller E, Rigo JM, Meyrand P, Branchereau P, Legendre P. Glycine release from radial cells modulates the spontaneous activity and its propagation during early spinal cord development. The Journal of Neuroscience. 2010;**30**:390-403

[17] Lonardoni D, Amin H, Di Marco S, Maccione A, Berdondini L, Nieus T. Recurrently connected and localized neuronal communities initiate coordinated spontaneous activity in neuronal networks. PLoS Computational Biology. 2017;**13**:e1005672

[18] Yu AC, Drejer J, Hertz L, Schousboe A. Pyruvate carboxylase activity in primary cultures of astrocytes and neurons. Journal of Neurochemistry. 1983;**41**:1484-1487

[19] Hertz L. The glutamate-glutamine (GABA) cycle: Importance of late postnatal development and potential reciprocal interactions between biosynthesis and degradation. Front Endocrinol (Lausanne). 2013;**4**:59

[20] Norenberg MD, Martinez-Hernandez A. Fine structural localization of glutamine synthetase in astrocytes of rat brain. Brain Research. 1979;**161**:303-310

[21] Chaudhry FA, Reimer RJ, Edwards RH. The glutamine commute: Take the N line and transfer to the A. The Journal of Cell Biology. 2002;**157**:349-355

[22] Hägglund MG, Sreedharan S, Nilsson VC, Shaik JH, Almkvist IM, Bäcklin S, Wrange O, Fredriksson R. Identification of SLC38A7 (SNAT7) protein as a glutamine transporter expressed in neurons. The Journal of Biological Chemistry. 2011;**286**:20500-20511

[23] Kvamme E, Torgner IA, Roberg B. Kinetics and localization of brain phosphate activated glutaminase. Journal of Neuroscience Research. 2001;**66**:951-958

[24] Hertz L, Peng L, Dienel GA. Energy metabolism in astrocytes: High rate of oxidative metabolism and spatiotemporal dependence on glycolysis/glycogenolysis. Journal of Cerebral Blood Flow and Metabolism. 2007;**27**:219-249

[25] Ottersen OP, Zhang N, Walberg F. Metabolic compartmentation of glutamate and glutamine: Morphological evidence obtained by quantitative immunocytochemistry in rat cerebellum. Neuroscience. 1992;**46**:519-534

[26] Omote H, Miyaji T, Juge N, Moriyama Y. Vesicular neurotransmitter transporter: Bioenergetics and regulation of glutamate transport. Biochemistry. 2011;**50**:5558-5565

[27] Rizzoli SO, Jahn R. Kiss-and-run, collapse and 'readily retrievable' vesicles. Traffic. 2007; **8**:1137-1144

[28] Traynelis SF, Wollmuth LP, McBain CJ, Menniti FS, Vance KM, Ogden KK, Hansen KB, Yuan H, Myers SJ, Dingledine R. Glutamate receptor ion channels: Structure, regulation, and function. Pharmacological Reviews. 2010;**62**:405-496

[29] Nowak L, Bregestovski P, Ascher P, Herbet A, Prochiantz A. Magnesium gates glutamate-activated channels in mouse central neurones. Nature. 1984;**307**:462-465

[30] Mayer ML, Westbrook GL, Guthrie PB. Voltage-dependent block by Mg^{2+} of NMDA responses in spinal cord neurones. Nature. 1984;**309**:261-263

[31] Pankratov Y, Lalo U. Calcium permeability of ligand-gated Ca^{2+} channels. European Journal of Pharmacology. 2014;**739**:60-73

[32] Collingridge GL, Kehl SJ, McLennan H. Excitatory amino acids in synaptic transmission in the Schaffer collateral-commissural pathway of the rat hippocampus. The Journal of Physiology. 1983;**334**:33-46

[33] Volianskis A, France G, Jensen MS, Bortolotto ZA, Jane DE, Collingridge GL. Long-term potentiation and the role of N-methyl-D-aspartate receptors. Brain Research. 2015;**1621**: 5-16

[34] Collingridge GL, Kehl SJ, Loo R, McLennan H. Effects of kainic and other amino acids on synaptic excitation in rat hippocampal slices: 1. Extracellular analysis. Experimental Brain Research. 1983;**52**:170-178

[35] Gnegy ME. Ca^{2+}/calmodulin signaling in NMDA-induced synaptic plasticity. Critical Reviews in Neurobiology. 2000;**14**:91-129

[36] Hebb DO. The Organization of Behavior. New York: Wiley & Sons; 1949

[37] Lisman J. A mechanism for the Hebb and the anti-Hebb processes underlying learning and memory. Proceedings of the National Academy of Sciences of the United States of America. 1989;**86**:9574-9578

[38] Carroll RC, Beattie EC, von Zastrow M, Malenka RC. Role of AMPA receptor endocytosis in synaptic plasticity. Nature Reviews. Neuroscience. 2001;**2**:315-324

[39] Niswender CM, Conn PJ. Metabotropic glutamate receptors: Physiology, pharmacology, and disease. Annual Review of Pharmacology and Toxicology. 2010;**50**:295-322

[40] Leaney JL, Milligan G, Tinker A. The G protein alpha subunit has a key role in determining the specificity of coupling to, but not the activation of, G protein-gated inwardly rectifying K(+) channels. The Journal of Biological Chemistry. 2000;**275**:921-929

[41] Sunahara RK, Taussig R. Isoforms of mammalian adenylyl cyclase: Multiplicities of signaling. Molecular Interventions. 2002;**2**:168-184

[42] Shigemoto R, Kinoshita A, Wada E, Nomura S, Ohishi H, Takada M, Flor PJ, Neki A, Abe T, Nakanishi S, Mizuno N. Differential presynaptic localization of metabotropic glutamate receptor subtypes in the rat hippocampus. The Journal of Neuroscience. 1997;**17**:7503-7522

[43] Danbolt NC. Glutamate uptake. Progress in Neurobiology. 2001;**65**:1-105

[44] Choi DW. Calcium and excitotoxic neuronal injury. Annals of the New York Academy of Sciences. 1994;**747**:162-171

[45] Kanai Y, Stelzner M, Nussberger S, Khawaja S, Hebert SC, Smith CP, Hediger MA. The neuronal and epithelial human high affinity glutamate transporter. Insights into structure and mechanism of transport. The Journal of Biological Chemistry. 1994;**269**:20599-20606

[46] Pomierny-Chamioło L, Rup K, Pomierny B, Niedzielska E, Kalivas PW, Filip M. Metabotropic glutamatergic receptors and their ligands in drug addiction. Pharmacology & Therapeutics. 2014;**142**:281-305

[47] Moran MM, McFarland K, Melendez RI, Kalivas PW, Seamans JK. Cystine/glutamate exchange regulates metabotropic glutamate receptor presynaptic inhibition of excitatory transmission and vulnerability to cocaine seeking. The Journal of Neuroscience. 2005;**25**:6389-6393

[48] Okada Y, Taniguchi H, Shimada C. High concentration of GABA and high glutamate decarboxylase activity in rat pancreatic islets and human insulinoma. Science. 1976;**194**: 620-622

[49] Jin H, Wu H, Osterhaus G, Wei J, Davis K, Sha D, Floor E, Hsu CC, Kopke RD, JY W. Demonstration of functional coupling between gamma-aminobutyric acid (GABA) synthesis and vesicular GABA transport into synaptic vesicles. Proceedings of the National Academy of Sciences of the United States of America. 2003;**100**:4293-4298

[50] Tian N, Petersen C, Kash S, Baekkeskov S, Copenhagen D, Nicoll R. The role of the synthetic enzyme GAD65 in the control of neuronal gamma-aminobutyric acid release. Proceedings of the National Academy of Sciences of the United States of America. 1999;**96**:12911-12916

[51] Baekkeskov S, Kanaani J. Palmitoylation cycles and regulation of protein function (review). Molecular Membrane Biology. 2009;**26**:42-54

[52] Rush DB, Leon RT, McCollum MH, Treu RW, Wei J. Palmitoylation and trafficking of GAD65 are impaired in a cellular model of Huntington's disease. The Biochemical Journal. 2012;**442**:39-48

[53] Bormann J. The 'ABC' of GABA receptors. Trends in Pharmacological Sciences. 2000; **21**:16-19

[54] Barnard EA, Skolnick P, Olsen RW, Mohler H, Sieghart W, Biggio G, Braestrup C, Bateson AN, Langer SZ. International Union of Pharmacology. XV. Subtypes of gamma-aminobutyric acidA receptors: Classification on the basis of subunit structure and receptor function. Pharmacological Reviews. 1998;**50**:291-313

[55] Sigel E, Steinmann ME. Structure, function, and modulation of GABA(A) receptors. The Journal of Biological Chemistry. 2012;**287**:40224-40231

[56] Brickley SG, Mody I. Extrasynaptic GABA(A) receptors: Their function in the CNS and implications for disease. Neuron. 2012;**73**:23-34

[57] Lüscher C, Slesinger PA. Emerging roles for G protein-gated inwardly rectifying potassium (GIRK) channels in health and disease. Nature Reviews. Neuroscience. 2010;**11**: 301-315

[58] Tedford HW, Zamponi GW. Direct G protein modulation of Cav2 calcium channels. Pharmacological Reviews. 2006;**58**:837-862

[59] Ong J, Kerr DI. Recent advances in GABAB receptors: From pharmacology to molecular biology. Acta Pharmacologica Sinica. 2000;**21**:111-123

[60] Davies CH, Starkey SJ, Pozza MF, Collingridge GL. GABA autoreceptors regulate the induction of LTP. Nature. 1991;**349**:609-611

[61] Schousboe A. Pharmacological and functional characterization of astrocytic GABA transport: A short review. Neurochemical Research. 2000;**25**:1241-1244

[62] Graus F, Titulaer MJ, Balu R, Benseler S, Bien CG, Cellucci T, Cortese I, Dale RC, Gelfand JM, Geschwind M, Glaser CA, Honnorat J, Höftberger R, Iizuka T, Irani SR, Lancaster E, Leypoldt F, Prüss H, Rae-Grant A, Reindl M, Rosenfeld MR, Rostásy K, Saiz A,

Venkatesan A, Vincent A, Wandinger KP, Waters P, Dalmau J. A clinical approach to diagnosis of autoimmune encephalitis. Lancet Neurology. 2016;**15**:391-404

[63] Dalmau J, Gleichman AJ, Hughes EG, Rossi JE, Peng X, Lai M, Dessain SK, Rosenfeld MR, Balice-Gordon R, Lynch DR. Anti-NMDA-receptor encephalitis: Case series and analysis of the effects of antibodies. Lancet Neurology. 2008;**7**:1091-1098

[64] Rogers SW, Andrews PI, Gahring LC, Whisenand T, Cauley K, Crain B, Hughes TE, Heinemann SF, McNamara JO. Autoantibodies to glutamate receptor GluR3 in Rasmussen's encephalitis. Science. 1994;**265**:648-651

[65] Dalmau J, Tüzün E, HY W, Masjuan J, Rossi JE, Voloschin A, Baehring JM, Shimazaki H, Koide R, King D, Mason W, Sansing LH, Dichter MA, Rosenfeld MR, Lynch DR. Paraneoplastic anti-N-methyl-D-aspartate receptor encephalitis associated with ovarian teratoma. Annals of Neurology. 2007;**61**:25-36

[66] Twyman RE, Gahring LC, Spiess J, Rogers SW. Glutamate receptor antibodies activate a subset of receptors and reveal an agonist binding site. Neuron. 1995;**14**:755-762

[67] Sillevis Smitt P, Kinoshita A, De Leeuw B, Moll W, Coesmans M, Jaarsma D, Henzen-Logmans S, Vecht C, De Zeeuw C, Sekiyama N, Nakanishi S, Shigemoto R. Paraneoplastic cerebellar ataxia due to autoantibodies against a glutamate receptor. The New England Journal of Medicine. 2000;**342**:21-27

[68] Jarius S, Wildemann B. 'Medusa-head ataxia': The expanding spectrum of Purkinje cell antibodies in autoimmune cerebellar ataxia. Part 1: Anti-mGluR1, anti-Homer-3, anti-Sj/ITPR1 and anti-CARP VIII. Journal of Neuroinflammation. 2015;**12**:166

[69] Hirai H, Launey T, Mikawa S, Torashima T, Yanagihara D, Kasaura T, Miyamoto A, Yuzaki M. New role of delta2-glutamate receptors in AMPA receptor trafficking and cerebellar function. Nature Neuroscience. 2003;**6**:869-876

[70] Guergueltcheva V, Azmanov DN, Angelicheva D, Smith KR, Chamova T, Florez L, Bynevelt M, Nguyen T, Cherninkova S, Bojinova V, Kaprelyan A, Angelova L, Morar B, Chandler D, Kaneva R, Bahlo M, Tournev I, Kalaydjieva L. Autosomal-recessive congenital cerebellar ataxia is caused by mutations in metabotropic glutamate receptor 1. American Journal of Human Genetics. 2012;**91**:553-564

[71] Massie A, Boillée S, Hewett S, Knackstedt L, Lewerenz J. Main path and byways: Non-vesicular glutamate release by system xc(−) as an important modifier of glutamatergic neurotransmission. Journal of Neurochemistry. 2015;**135**:1062-1079

[72] Anderson CM, Swanson RA. Astrocyte glutamate transport: Review of properties, regulation, and physiological functions. Glia. 2000;**32**:1-14

[73] Fujikawa DG. The role of excitotoxic programmed necrosis in acute brain injury. Computational and Structural Biotechnology Journal. 2015;**13**:212-221

[74] Lewerenz J, Maher P. Chronic glutamate toxicity in neurodegenerative diseases-what is the evidence? Frontiers in Neuroscience. 2015;**9**:469

[75] Höftberger R, Titulaer MJ, Sabater L, Dome B, Rózsás A, Hegedus B, Hoda MA, Laszlo V, Ankersmit HJ, Harms L, Boyero S, de Felipe A, Saiz A, Dalmau J, Graus F. Encephalitis and GABAB receptor antibodies: Novel findings in a new case series of 20 patients. Neurology. 2013;**81**:1500-1506

[76] Honnorat J, Saiz A, Giometto B, Vincent A, Brieva L, de Andres C, Maestre J, Fabien N, Vighetto A, Casamitjana R, Thivolet C, Tavolato B, Antoine J, Trouillas P, Graus F. Cerebellar ataxia with anti-glutamic acid decarboxylase antibodies: Study of 14 patients. Archives of Neurology. 2001;**58**:225-230

[77] Mitoma H, Ishida K, Shizuka-Ikeda M, Mizusawa H. Dual impairment of GABAA- and GABAB-receptor-mediated synaptic responses by autoantibodies to glutamic acid decarboxylase. Journal of the Neurological Sciences. 2003;**208**:51-56

[78] Ishida K, Mitoma H, Song SY, Uchihara T, Inaba A, Eguchi S, Kobayashi T, Mizusawa H. Selective suppression of cerebellar GABAergic transmission by an autoantibody to glutamic acid decarboxylase. Annals of Neurology. 1999;**46**:263-267

[79] Manto MU, Laute MA, Aguera M, Rogemond V, Pandolfo M, Honnorat J. Effects of anti-glutamic acid decarboxylase antibodies associated with neurological diseases. Annals of Neurology. 2007;**61**:544-551

[80] Manto MU, Hampe CS, Rogemond V, Honnorat J. Respective implications of glutamate decarboxylase antibodies in stiff person syndrome and cerebellar ataxia. Orphanet Journal of Rare Diseases. 2011;**6**:3

[81] Hampe CS, Petrosini L, De Bartolo P, Caporali P, Cutuli D, Laricchiuta D, Foti F, Radtke JR, Vidova V, Honnorat J, Manto M. Monoclonal antibodies to 65kDa glutamate decarboxylase induce epitope specific effects on motor and cognitive functions in rats. Orphanet Journal of Rare Diseases. 2013;**8**:82

[82] Manto M, Honnorat J, Hampe CS, Guerra-Narbona R, Lopez-Ramos JC, Delgado-Garcia JM, Saitow F, Suzuki H, Yanagawa Y, Mizusawa H, Mitoma H. Disease-specific monoclonal antibodies targeting glutamate decarboxylase impair GABAergic neurotransmission and affect motor learning and behavioral functions. Frontiers in Behavioral Neuroscience. 2015;**9**:78

[83] Dinkel K, Meinck H, Jury KM, Karges W, Richter W. Inhibition of gamma-aminobutyric acid synthesis by glutamic acid decarboxylase autoantibodies in stiff-man syndrome. Annals of Neurology. 1998;**44**:194-201

[84] Hansen N, Grunewald B, Weishaupt A, Colaco MN, Toyka KV, Sommer C, Geis C. Human Stiff person syndrome IgG-containing high-titer anti-GAD65 autoantibodies induce motor dysfunction in rats. Experimental Neurology. 2013;**239**:202-209

[85] Ishida K, Mitoma H, Mizusawa H. Reversibility of cerebellar GABAergic synapse impairment induced by anti-glutamic acid decarboxylase autoantibodies. Journal of the Neurological Sciences. 2008;**271**:186-190

[86] Hill KE, Clawson SA, Rose JW, Carlson NG, Greenlee JE. Cerebellar Purkinje cells incorporate immunoglobulins and immunotoxins in vitro: Implications for human neurological disease and immunotherapeutics. Journal of Neuroinflammation. 2009;**6**:31

[87] Mitoma H, Manto M, Hampe CS: Pathogenic roles of glutamic acid decarboxylase 65 autoantibodies in cerebellar ataxias. Journal of Immunology Research 2017;**2017**: 2913297.

[88] Wong WT, Wang M, Li W. Regulation of microglia by ionotropic glutamatergic and GABAergic neurotransmission. Neuron Glia Biology. 2011;**7**:41-46

[89] Olmos G, Lladó J. Tumor necrosis factor alpha: A link between neuroinflammation and excitotoxicity. Mediators of Inflammation. 2014;**2014**:861231

[90] Ishida K, Mitoma H, Wada Y, Oka T, Shibahara J, Saito Y, Murayama S, Mizusawa H. Selective loss of Purkinje cells in a patient with anti-glutamic acid decarboxylase antibody-associated cerebellar ataxia. Journal of Neurology, Neurosurgery and Psychiatry. 2007;**78**: 190-192

[91] Erdö SL, Wolff JR. Gamma-aminobutyric acid outside the mammalian brain. Journal of Neurochemistry. 1990;**54**:363-372

[92] Woods SC, Lutz TA, Geary N, Langhans W. Pancreatic signals controlling food intake; insulin, glucagon and amylin. Philosophical Transactions of the Royal Society of London. Series B, Biological Sciences. 2006;**361**:1219-1235

[93] Gromada J, Franklin I, Wollheim CB. Alpha-cells of the endocrine pancreas: 35 years of research but the enigma remains. Endocrine Reviews. 2007;**28**:84-116

[94] MacDonald MJ. Influence of glucose on pyruvate carboxylase expression in pancreatic islets. Archives of Biochemistry and Biophysics. 1995;**319**:128-132

[95] Hayashi M, Morimoto R, Yamamoto A, Moriyama Y. Expression and localization of vesicular glutamate transporters in pancreatic islets, upper gastrointestinal tract, and testis. The Journal of Histochemistry and Cytochemistry. 2003;**51**:1375-1390

[96] Thomas-Reetz A, Hell JW, During MJ, Walch-Solimena C, Jahn R, De Camilli P. A g-aminobutyric acid transporter driven by a proton pump is present in synaptic-like microvewsicles of pancreatic ß cells. Proceedings of the National Academy of Sciences. 1993;**90**:5317-5321

[97] Braun M, Ramracheya R, Bengtsson M, Clark A, Walker JN, Johnson PR, Rorsman P. Gamma-aminobutyric acid (GABA) is an autocrine excitatory transmitter in human pancreatic beta-cells. Diabetes. 2010;**59**:1694-1701

[98] Gammelsaeter R, Frøyland M, Aragón C, Danbolt NC, Fortin D, Storm-Mathisen J, Davanger S, Gundersen V. Glycine, GABA and their transporters in pancreatic islets of Langerhans: Evidence for a paracrine transmitter interplay. Journal of Cell Science. 2004;**117**:3749-3758

[99] Vincent ST, Hökfelt T, J-Y W, Eide RP, Morgan LM, Kimmel JR. Immunohistochemical studies of the GABA system in the pancreas. Neuroendocrinology. 1983;**36**:197-204

[100] Garry DJ, Appel NM, Garry MG, Sorenson RL. Cellular and subcellular immunolocalization of L-glutamate decarboxylase in rat pancreatic islets. Journal of Histochemistry & Cytochemistry. 1988;**36**:573-580

[101] Reetz A, Solimena M, Matteoli M, Folli F, Takei K, De Camilli P. GABA and pancreatic β-cells: Co-localization of glutamic acid decarboxylase (GAD) and GABA with synaptic-like microvesicles suggests their role in GABA storage and secretion. The EMBO Journal. 1991;**10**:1275-1284

[102] Kanaani J, Lissin D, Kash SF, Baekkeskov S. The hydrophilic isoform of glutamate decarboxylase, GAD67, is targeted to membranes and nerve terminals independent of dimerization with the hydrophobic membrane-anchored isoform, GAD65. The Journal of Biological Chemistry. 1999;**274**:37200-37209

[103] Rorsman P, Berggren PO, Bokvist K, Ericson H, Möhler H, Östensson CG, Smith PA. Glucose-inhibition of glucagon secretion involves activation of GABAA-receptor chloride channels. Nature. 1989;**341**:233-236

[104] Winnock F, Ling Z, De Proft R, Dejonghe S, Schuit F, Gorus F, Pipeleers D. Correlation between GABA release from rat islet beta-cells and their metabolic state. American Journal of Physiology. Endocrinology and Metabolism. 2002;**282**:E937-E942

[105] von Blankenfeld G, Turner J, Ahnert-Hilger G, John M, Enkvist MO, Stephenson F, Kettenmann H, Wiedenmann B: Expression of functional GABAA receptors in neuroendocrine gastropancreatic cells. Pflügers Archiv 1995;**430**:381-388

[106] Braun M, Wendt A, Birnir B, Broman J, Eliasson L, Galvanovskis J, Gromada J, Mulder H, Rorsman P. Regulated exocytosis of GABA-containing synaptic-like microvesicles in pancreatic beta-cells. The Journal of General Physiology. 2004;**123**:191-204

[107] Soltani N, Qiu H, Aleksic M, Glinka Y, Zhao F, Liu R, Li Y, Zhang N, Chakrabarti R, Ng T, Jin T, Zhang H, Lu WY, Feng ZP, Prud'homme GJ, Wang Q. GABA exerts protective and regenerative effects on islet beta cells and reverses diabetes. Proceedings of the National Academy of Sciences of the United States of America. 2011;**108**:11692-11697

[108] Smismans A, Schuit F, Pipeleers D. Nutrient regulation of gamma-aminobutyric acid release from islet beta cells. Diabetologia. 1997;**40**:1411-1415

[109] Brice NL, Varadi A, Ashcroft SJ, Molnar E. Metabotropic glutamate and GABA(B) receptors contribute to the modulation of glucose-stimulated insulin secretion in pancreatic beta cells. Diabetologia. 2002;**45**:242-252

[110] Sorenson RL, Garry DG, Brelje TC. Structural and functional considerations of GABA in islets of Langerhans. Beta-cells and nerves. Diabetes. 1991;**40**:1365-1374

[111] Xu E, Kumar M, Zhang Y, Ju W, Obata T, Zhang N, Liu S, Wendt A, Deng S, Ebina Y, Wheeler MB, Braun M, Wang Q. Intra-islet insulin suppresses glucagon release via GABA-GABAA receptor system. Cell Metabolism. 2006;**3**:47-58

[112] Franklin I, Gromada J, Gjinovci A, Theander S, Wollheim CB. Beta-cell secretory products activate alpha-cell ATP-dependent potassium channels to inhibit glucagon release. Diabetes. 2005;**54**:1808-1815

[113] Zhang Q, Ramracheya R, Lahmann C, Tarasov A, Bengtsson M, Braha O, Braun M, Brereton M, Collins S, Galvanovskis J, Gonzalez A, Groschner LN, Rorsman NJ, Salehi A, Travers ME, Walker JN, Gloyn AL, Gribble F, Johnson PR, Reimann F, Ashcroft FM, Rorsman P. Role of KATP channels in glucose-regulated glucagon secretion and impaired counterregulation in type 2 diabetes. Cell Metabolism. 2013;**18**:871-882

[114] Wendt A, Birnir B, Buschard K, Gromada J, Salehi A, Sewing S, Rorsman P, Braun M. Glucose inhibition of glucagon secretion from rat alpha-cells is mediated by GABA released from neighboring beta-cells. Diabetes. 2004;**53**:1038-1045

[115] Ostenson CG. Regulation of glucagon release: Effects of insulin on the pancreatic A2-cell of the guinea pig. Diabetologia. 1979;**17**:325-330

[116] Gonoi T, Mizuno N, Inagaki N, Kuromi H, Seino Y, Miyazaki J, Seino S. Functional neuronal ionotropic glutamate receptors are expressed in the non-neuronal cell line MIN6. The Journal of Biological Chemistry. 1994;**269**:16989-16992

[117] Cabrera O, Jacques-Silva MC, Speier S, Yang SN, Köhler M, Fachado A, Vieira E, Zierath JR, Kibbey R, Berman DM, Kenyon NS, Ricordi C, Caicedo A, Berggren PO. Glutamate is a positive autocrine signal for glucagon release. Cell Metabolism. 2008;**7**:545-554

[118] Storto M, Capobianco L, Battaglia G, Molinaro G, Gradini R, Riozzi B, Di Mambro A, Mitchell KJ, Bruno V, Vairetti MP, Rutter GA, Nicoletti F. Insulin secretion is controlled by mGlu5 metabotropic glutamate receptors. Molecular Pharmacology. 2006;**69**:1234-1241

[119] Uehara S, Muroyama A, Echigo N, Morimoto R, Otsuka M, Yatsushiro S, Moriyama Y. Metabotropic glutamate receptor type 4 is involved in autoinhibitory cascade for glucagon secretion by alpha-cells of islet of Langerhans. Diabetes. 2004;**53**:998-1006

[120] Bertrand G, Puech R, Loubatieres-Mariani MM, Bockaert J. Glutamate stimulates insulin secretion and improves glucose tolerance in rats. The American Journal of Physiology. 1995;**269**:E551-E556

[121] Otter S, Lammert E. Exciting times for pancreatic islets: Glutamate signaling in endocrine cells. Trends in Endocrinology and Metabolism. 2016;**27**:177-188

[122] Di Cairano ES, Davalli AM, Perego L, Sala S, Sacchi VF, La Rosa S, Finzi G, Placidi C, Capella C, Conti P, Centonze VE, Casiraghi F, Bertuzzi F, Folli F, Perego C. The glial glutamate transporter 1 (GLT1) is expressed by pancreatic beta-cells and prevents glutamate-induced beta-cell death. The Journal of Biological Chemistry. 2011;**286**:14007-14018

[123] McCrimmon R. The mechanisms that underlie glucose sensing during hypoglycaemia in diabetes. Diabetic Medicine. 2008;**25**:513-522

[124] Fukuda M, Tanaka A, Tahara Y, Ikegami H, Yamamoto Y, Kumahara Y, Shima K. Correlation between minimal secretory capacity of pancreatic beta-cells and stability of diabetic control. Diabetes. 1988;**37**:81-88

[125] Müller WA, Faloona GR, Unger RH. Hyperglucagonemia in diabetic ketoacidosis. Its prevalence and significance. American Journal of Medicine. 1973;**54**:52-57

[126] Reaven GM, Chen YD, Golay A, Swislocki AL, Jaspan JB. Documentation of hyperglucagonemia throughout the day in nonobese and obese patients with noninsulin-dependent diabetes mellitus. The Journal of Clinical Endocrinology and Metabolism. 1987;**64**:106-110

[127] Perry T, Haughey NJ, Mattson MP, Egan JM, Greig NH. Protection and reversal of excitotoxic neuronal damage by glucagon-like peptide-1 and exendin-4. The Journal of Pharmacology and Experimental Therapeutics. 2002;**302**:881-888

[128] Perry T, Greig NH. The glucagon-like peptides: A new genre in therapeutic targets for intervention in Alzheimer's disease. Journal of Alzheimer's Disease. 2002;**4**:487-496

[129] Rosenstock J, Hollander P, Gadde KM, Sun X, Strauss R, Leung A, Group O-S. A randomized, double-blind, placebo-controlled, multicenter study to assess the efficacy and safety of topiramate controlled release in the treatment of obese type 2 diabetic patients. Diabetes Care. 2007;**30**:1480-1486

[130] Davalli AM, Perego C, Folli FB, Bosi E. Long-lasting remission of type 1 diabetes following treatment with topiramate for generalized seizures. Acta Diabetologica. 2012; **49**:75-79

[131] Wan Y, Wang Q, Prud'homme GJ. GABAergic system in the endocrine pancreas: A new target for diabetes treatment. Diabetes, Metabolic Syndrome and Obesity. 2015;**8**:79-87

[132] Alam S, Laughton DL, Walding A, Wolstenholme AJ. Human peripheral blood mononuclear cells express GABAA receptor subunits. Molecular Immunology. 2006;**43**:1432-1442

[133] Mendu SK, Bhandage A, Jin Z, Birnir B. Different subtypes of GABA-A receptors are expressed in human, mouse and rat T lymphocytes. PLoS One. 2012;**7**:e42959

[134] Tian J, Chau C, Hales TG, Kaufman DL. GABA(A) receptors mediate inhibition of T cell responses. Journal of Neuroimmunology. 1999;**96**:21-28

[135] Ligon B, Yang J, Morin SB, Ruberti MF, Steer ML. Regulation of pancreatic islet cell survival and replication by gamma-aminobutyric acid. Diabetologia. 2007;**50**:764-773

[136] Tian J, Dang H, Chen Z, Guan A, Jin Y, Atkinson MA, Kaufman DL. gamma-Aminobutyric acid regulates both the survival and replication of human beta-cells. Diabetes. 2013;**62**: 3760-3765

[137] Thorel F, Népote V, Avril I, Kohno K, Desgraz R, Chera S, Herrera PL. Conversion of adult pancreatic alpha-cells to beta-cells after extreme beta-cell loss. Nature. 2010;**464**: 1149-1154

[138] Ben-Othman N, Vieira A, Courtney M, Record F, Gjernes E, Avolio F, Hadzic B, Druelle N, Napolitano T, Navarro-Sanz S, Silvano S, Al-Hasani K, Pfeifer A, Lacas-Gervais S, Leuckx G, Marroquí L, Thévenet J, Madsen OD, Eizirik DL, Heimberg H, Kerr-Conte J,

Pattou F, Mansouri A, Collombat P. Long-term GABA administration induces alpha cell-mediated beta-like cell neogenesis. Cell. 2017;**168**:73-85 e11

[139] Rutter GA. GABA signaling: A route to new pancreatic β cells. Cell Research. 2017;**27**: 309-310

[140] Bansal P, Wang S, Liu S, Xiang YY, WY L, Wang Q. GABA coordinates with insulin in regulating secretory function in pancreatic INS-1 β-cells. PLoS One. 2011;**6**:e26225

[141] Bailey SJ, Ravier MA, Rutter GA. Glucose-dependent regulation of gamma-aminobutyric acid (GABA A) receptor expression in mouse pancreatic islet alpha-cells. Diabetes. 2007; **56**:320-327

Chapter 6

Antagonists of Ionotropic Receptors for the Inhibitory Neurotransmitter GABA: Therapeutic Indications

Tina Hinton and Graham A. R. Johnston

Additional information is available at the end of the chapter

http://dx.doi.org/10.5772/intechopen.72678

Abstract

Agents that antagonize the action of GABA on ionotropic receptors are widely used to probe the function of this neurotransmitter. Three such agents are in common use: bicuculline, gabazine, and picrotoxinin. These three agents produce convulsions on systemic administration but act in significantly different ways. Bicuculline is a competitive antagonist of $GABA_A$ receptors. Gabazine is also a competitive antagonist of $GABA_A$ receptors, interacting with different residues on the receptors. Picrotoxinin is a noncompetitive antagonist acting on the chloride channel of $GABA_A$ and several other ionotropic CYS-loop receptors including glycine, $GABA_C$, and 5-HT_3 receptors. Many other structurally diverse agents are now known to act as GABA receptor antagonists, providing opportunities for the discovery of agents with selectivity for the myriad of ionotropic GABA receptors. TPMPA is a selective antagonist for $GABA_C$ receptors, which are insensitive to bicuculline. Like TPMPA, many antagonists of ionotropic GABA receptors are not convulsants, indicating that there is still much to be learnt about GABA function in the brain from the study of such agents and their possible therapeutic uses. The most recently discovered $GABA_A$ receptor nonconvulsive antagonist is S44819, which is subtype selective for α5-containing receptors, and is arousing much interest in relation to cognition.

Keywords: antagonists, GABA receptors, bicuculline, gabazine, picrotoxinin

1. Introduction

"Advantages of an Antagonist" headed the Nature editorial in 1970 on the paper reporting the antagonist action of the convulsant alkaloid bicuculline on receptors for the neurotransmitter GABA in the cat spinal cord [1, 2]. The editorial predicted "With this tool it should now be possible to map fairly rapidly the distribution of GABA-inhibitory synapses in the CNS, and to determine whether they are as numerous and widely distributed as the relatively high GABA content of the tissue would suggest." Indeed, interest in GABA antagonists continues today, with more than 120 publications per year containing the terms "bicuculline" and "GABA" since 1970 [3]. GABA-inhibitory synapses are widely distributed in the CNS with GABA being released by up to 40% of neurons in many brain regions [4]. Specific GABA receptor antagonists have been described as "essential tools of physiological and pharmacological elucidation of the different types of GABA receptor inhibition" [5].

GABA receptors can be divided into two major types based on their mechanism of action dating from the studies by David Hill and Norman Bowery in 1981 on the binding of the GABA analog baclofen to rat brain membranes [6]. They described a receptor that "differs from the classical GABA site as it is unaffected by recognized GABA antagonists such as bicuculline." They went on to state "We propose to designate the classical site as the $GABA_A$ and the novel site as the $GABA_B$ receptor." We now know that $GABA_A$ receptors are ionotropic receptors and that $GABA_B$ receptors are metabotropic. This perspective on GABA receptor antagonists is limited to mammalian ionotropic receptors.

Ionotropic GABA receptors are ligand-gated ion channels, where binding of GABA necessitates a change in conformation, which leads to opening of the ion channel. The ion channel is permeable to chloride, and increased conductance of this anion stabilizes the membrane potential, thereby reducing excitatory depolarization of the postsynaptic membrane. On the other hand, metabotropic GABA receptors are G-protein-coupled receptors, where GABA binding activates a variety of second messengers that lead to closing of cation channels to prevent sodium and calcium entry and opening of potassium channels to permit potassium efflux. The net effect is a reduction in excitability of the pre- or postsynaptic cell.

Ionotropic GABA receptors are part of the CYS-loop group of receptors that include glycine and $5\text{-}HT_3$ receptors. Ionotropic GABA receptors may be divided into two classes based on their sensitivity to antagonists. $GABA_A$ receptors may be antagonized selectively by bicuculline, while $GABA_C$ receptors are antagonized selectively by TPMPA ((1,2,5,6-tetrahydropyridin-4-yl)methylphosphinic acid) and are insensitive to bicuculline [7]. It turns out that these two classes differ in several other respects. While $GABA_C$ receptors are relatively simple homomeric pentameric receptors, $GABA_A$ receptors are complex heteromeric pentameric receptors consisting of a variety of protein subunits, resulting in different possible combinations and thus a myriad of receptor subtypes. The structural complexity of the $GABA_A$ receptors further supports a range of allosteric binding sites which are binding targets for endogenous and exogenous allosteric modulators of these receptors. For example, receptors containing α_1, α_2, α_3, or α_5 subunits along with a γ_{2L} subunit permit high-affinity benzodiazepine binding [8]. Barbiturates are known to bind to an allosteric site on all $GABA_A$ receptor subtypes [9]. As another example, receptors containing δ subunits are targets for endogenous neurosteroids and ethanol [10–12]. Development of subtype-selective agonists, antagonists, and modulators of the ionotropic GABA receptors is imperative to the provision of valuable experimental tools for elucidation of the distribution and various functions of these $GABA_A$ receptor subtypes.

Antagonism of ionotropic GABA receptors may result from three distinct mechanisms: competitive antagonism where the binding site for the drug may overlap with the GABA-binding

http://dx.doi.org/10.5772/intechopen.72678

site, i.e., the orthosteric site; negative allosteric modulation where the drug binds to a site distinct from the orthosteric site to reduce the affinity of the agonist; and noncompetitive antagonism where the drug binds to a site on the chloride channel to reduce chloride permeability or channel opening by GABA [13]. In this perspective, we consider examples of all three types of antagonism of the ionotropic GABA receptors.

2. Picrotoxin, a channel blocker of ionotropic GABA receptors

The first reported GABA receptor antagonist was picrotoxin, a convulsant plant product, a combination of the Greek words "picros" (bitter) and "toxicon" (poison). It is a 50:50 mixture of picrotoxinin (**Figure 1**) and picrotin with picrotoxinin being the more active component as a GABA receptor antagonist. Early reports showed that picrotoxin antagonized the action of GABA at invertebrate inhibitory synapses and that it reduced presynaptic inhibition in the spinal cord [14]. In 1968, Davidoff and Aprison showed that picrotoxin antagonized the inhibitory

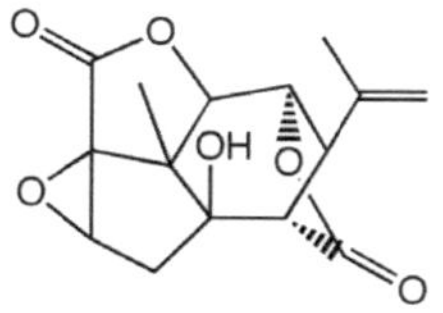

Picrotoxinin
$GABA_A$, $GABA_C$, $5HT_3$
non-competitive antagonist

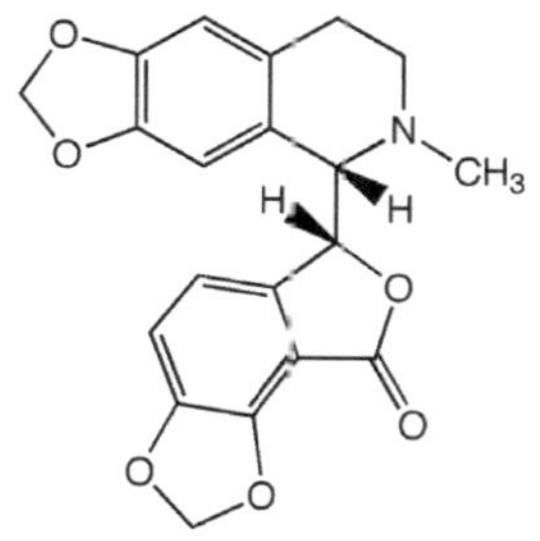

Bicuculline
$GABA_A$ competitive antagonist

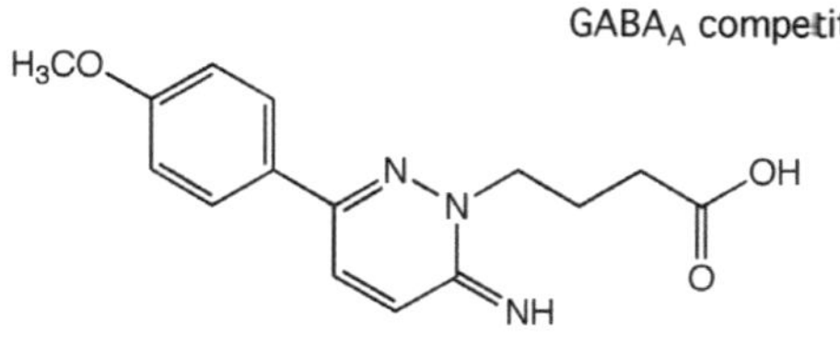

Gabazine (SR 95531)
$GABA_A$ competitive antagonist

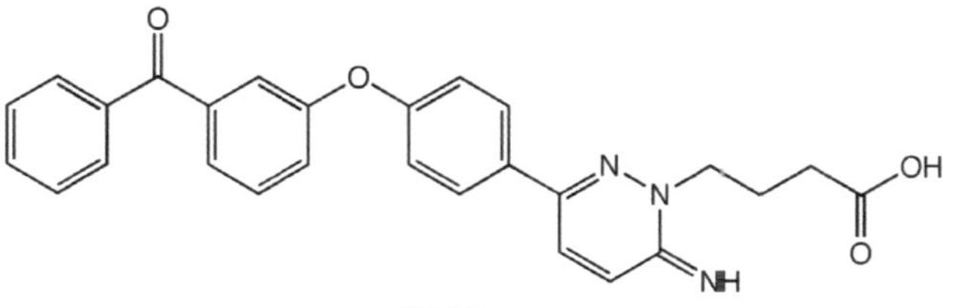

GZ-B1
Photo-activated antagonist

Figure 1. $GABA_A$ receptor antagonists that are convulsants.

action of glycine on spinal neurones [15]. Curtis et al. [16] reported antagonist action against both glycine and GABA, but the results were inconsistent due to the lack of ionization using the microiontophoresis method of drug administration.

These technical difficulties were eventually overcome using recombinant receptors with bath application of picrotoxin showing it to be a mixed/noncompetitive $GABA_A$ receptor antagonist [17]. But picrotoxin was also shown to be an antagonist of other CYS-loop receptors, including glycine, $GABA_C$, and $5\text{-}HT_3$ receptors [18]. Thus, the utility of picrotoxin (and also picrotoxinin) as an experimental tool is mitigated by its lack of selectivity for $GABA_A$ receptors. It also has no therapeutic potential owing to its potent convulsant effects.

Many terpenoids related to picrotoxinin are convulsants acting on ionotropic receptors for GABA and glycine [19]. Of particular interest is tutin that occurs in the berries and flowers of the indigenous New Zealand tutu plant, *Coriaria arborea*, and has been credited with convulsing a circus elephant that consumed the berries [20]. Toxic honey was also produced from bees that collected nectar from the flowers.

3. Bicuculline, a competitive antagonist of $GABA_A$ receptors

The discovery of bicuculline as a selective antagonist of what became known as $GABA_A$ receptors arose out of a systematic study of convulsant alkaloids [3]. It was well known that the most widely understood convulsant alkaloid, strychnine, antagonized the inhibitory action of glycine without influencing the inhibitory action of GABA [21]. Indeed, most convulsant alkaloids turned out to be glycine receptor antagonists with the important exception of bicuculline (**Figure 1**), an alkaloid from *Dicentra cucullaria* [22].

While bicuculline is selective for $GABA_A$ receptors, having little effect on $GABA_B$, $GABA_C$, glycine, and $5\text{-}HT_3$ receptors, its action is largely independent of $GABA_A$ subunit composition [17, 23]. Selectivity for $GABA_A$ receptors makes bicuculline a powerful experimental tool but without any therapeutic potential owing to the nonselective nature of binding to all $GABA_A$ receptor subtypes, causing profound convulsive effects. Bicuculline binds at the orthosteric site to stabilize the receptor in a closed state. It is three times the size of GABA and thus is able to bind to sites on the receptor that GABA cannot reach [3]. Bicuculline acts as a competitive antagonist in which it competitively inhibits GABA agonist binding to $GABA_A$ receptors, and GABA competitively inhibits bicuculline binding [24]. Single channel studies show that by competing with GABA for its binding site, bicuculline acts to reduce both chloride channel open time and opening frequency [25].

At physiological pH, bicuculline is slowly converted to bicucine, a much less active convulsant [26]. This transformation is slowly reversed at acidic pH. Thus, bicuculline solutions should always be freshly prepared in order to preserve maximum convulsant potency. Quaternary salts of bicuculline, such as bicuculline methiodide ("N-methyl bicuculline") or methochloride, are much more stable than bicuculline, are more water soluble, and are of similar potency as GABA receptor antagonists, but they do not cross the blood-brain barrier on systemic administration [27, 28]. The quaternary salts differ in their pharmacology to bicuculline itself in that they are much less selective. It is not always clear in publications whether the investigators use bicuculline or a quaternary salt [3]. The quaternary salts have significant actions on nicotinic receptors, calcium-activated potassium channels, and acetylcholinesterase [29–31]. Thus, while ensuring chemical stability of bicuculline, the quaternary salts may be less effective tools owing to their reduced binding specificity for $GABA_A$ receptors. Subject to these considerations, bicuculline and its quaternary salts continue to be used extensively as $GABA_A$ receptor antagonists in experimentation.

Extensive structure-activity studies have been carried out on bicuculline with little improvement on potency, selectivity, or stability [3]. Investigations of bicuculline analogs devoid of the phenyl ring fused to the lactone moiety have yielded positive allosteric modulators. These analogs do not bind to the orthosteric binding site on $GABA_A$ receptors. Instead, they bind to the high-affinity benzodiazepine site on $GABA_A$ receptor subtypes containing subunit combinations described above and show subtype selectivity that differs from that shown by benzodiazepines [32].

Bicuculline has been shown to improve special memory in the rat hippocampus [33].

4. Gabazine, a competitive antagonist of $GABA_A$ receptors

Gabazine (also known as SR 95531, **Figure 1**) resulted from a study of arylaminopyridazine analogs of GABA. It was found to be a relatively specific, potent, and competitive antagonist of $GABA_A$ receptors [34]. Although both are functionally competitive inhibitors, gabazine and bicuculline also interact with other residues on $GABA_A$ receptors [35, 36]. Neither gabazine nor bicuculline compete for the binding at the barbiturate or neurosteroid binding sites on $GABA_A$ receptors. It is suggested that both antagonists act "as allosteric inhibitors of channel opening for the $GABA_A$ receptor after binding to the GABA-binding site" [36]. Gabazine has little activity at $GABA_C$ receptors [37]. At binary β3δ recombinant $GABA_A$ receptors, gabazine antagonized GABA currents, whereas bicuculline activated these receptors [38]. Thus, while functioning as competitive antagonists for $GABA_A$ receptors, gabazine and bicuculline clearly interact with different residues on $GABA_A$ receptors.

Structural analogs of gabazine have identified more potent agents [39]. Gabazine analogs incorporating photoactive groups, such as GZ-B1 (**Figure 1**), have been developed as photo-activated antagonists of $GABA_A$ receptors [40]. These antagonists provide dynamic tools for visualizing $GABA_A$ receptors, permitting a novel means of investigating receptor location, function, and trafficking [40].

5. TPMPA and related compounds, competitive antagonists of $GABA_C$ receptors

$GABA_C$ receptors, also known as GABA-ρ and $GABA_A$-ρ receptors, have distinctive distribution and pharmacological properties to $GABA_A$ receptors, making them particularly interesting [41].

They are CYS-loop ligand-gated ion channels with a similar pentameric structure to GABA$_A$ receptors but are not so widely distributed. They are homomeric rather than heteromeric and therefore much simpler receptors. These properties make them important drug targets [42].

TPMPA ((1,2,5,6-Tetrahydropyridin-4-yl)methylphosphinic acid, **Figure 2**) was the first selective GABA$_C$ receptor antagonist to be synthesized [43, 44]. Other GABA$_C$ receptor antagonists include the bicyclic GABA analog, THIP (Gaboxadol, 4,5,6,7-**t**etra**h**ydro**i**soxazolo(5,4-c)**p**yridin-3-ol, **Figure 2**), which is a moderately potent antagonist at the GABA$_C$ receptors, yet a potent agonist at GABA$_A$ receptor receptors [45]. Aza-THIP (1H,4H,5H,6H,7H-pyrazolo[3,4-c]pyridin-3-ol) is inactive at GABA$_A$ receptors but shows moderately potent antagonism at GABA$_C$ receptors. Phosphinic, phosphonic, and seleninic analogs of isonipecotic acid have also been shown to act as selective GABA$_C$ receptor antagonists [46], as have amide and hydroxamate analogs of 4-aminocyclopent-1-enecarboxylic acid [47].

Unlike many GABA$_A$ receptor antagonists, TPMPA is not a convulsant, consistent with many instances that GABA$_A$ and GABA$_C$ receptors have been shown to mediate opposing functions, for example, on excitability [48] and in memory formation [49].

TPMPA and other GABA$_C$ receptor antagonists have been used to demonstrate the important role of GABA$_C$ receptors in many aspects of vision [50–53]. TPMPA was shown to inhibit

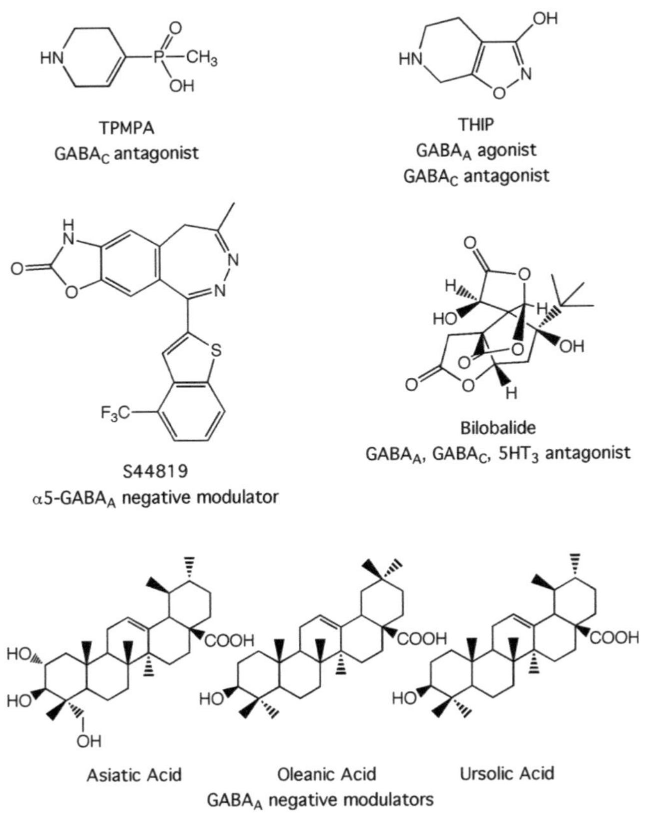

Figure 2. GABA$_A$ receptor antagonists that are not convulsants.

http://dx.doi.org/10.5772/intechopen.72678

form-deprivation myopia [51], while (3-aminopropyl)-n-butylphosphinic acid (CGP36742 or SGS742) was found to inhibit the development of myopia in chicks [50]. Thus, TPMPA and related $GABA_C$ receptor antagonists have been suggested for the treatment of myopia, administered intravitreally, orally, and ophthalmically [52]. Indeed, $GABA_C$ receptor antagonists have been patented for the treatment of myopia [52].

$GABA_C$ receptor antagonists have also been useful experimental tools for demonstrating a role for these receptors in learning and memory [49, 50, 54]. TPMPA and the structural analog P4MPA ((piperidin-4-yl)methylphosphinic acid) were shown to enhance short-term memory in a bead discrimination task following injection into the multimodal association forebrain area in chicks [49]. Injection of bicuculline caused the opposite effect. TPMPA has also been used to demonstrate a role for $GABA_C$ receptors in fear learning and memory in rats [54]. Rats administered TPMPA via bilateral cannulae injections into the lateral amygdala showed reduced freezing in a foot shock conditioned fear task. This reduction in fear learning and memory is likely mediated by presynaptically located $GABA_C$ receptors in the lateral amygdala [54].

Arising out of studies on the orally active $GABA_{(B/C)}$ receptor antagonist (3-aminopropyl)-n-butylphosphinic acid (CGP36742 or SGS742) [55], *cis*- and *trans*-(3-aminocyclopentanyl) butylphosphinic acid were found to be selective potent $GABA_C$ receptor antagonists that enhanced learning and memory in rats in the Morris water maze task [50].

Based on the structure of the selective $GABA_C$ receptor antagonist (*S*)-4-ACPBPA [(4-aminocyclopenten-1-yl)-butylphosphinic acid], a series of fluorescent ligands were produced linking fluorophores to the parent compound [56]. One of these fluorescent ligands, (*S*)-4-ACPBPA-C5-BODIPY, showed moderately potent antagonism for $GABA_C$ receptors with greater than 100 times selectivity for these receptors over $GABA_A$ receptors. (*S*)-4-ACPBPA-C5-BODIPY thus provides a valuable molecular probe for the role of $GABA_C$ receptors in physiological and pathological processes [56].

6. Bilobalide, a nonconvulsant channel blocker

Bilobalide (**Figure 2**) and a series of terpenoids known as ginkgolides isolated from *Ginkgo biloba* are structurally related to picrotoxinin and are relatively potent $GABA_A$ and $GABA_C$ receptor antagonists [57], but they also act on glycine and 5-HT_3 receptors [58, 59].

Unlike picrotoxin, bilobalide is an anticonvulsant. This may be due to its potent action on $GABA_C$ receptors [57]. Bilobalide also has differing effects to those of picrotoxin on the modulation of $GABA_A$ receptors by structurally different modulators [60], suggesting a different binding profile to picrotoxin to negatively modulate the $GABA_A$ receptors.

Thus, there are $GABA_A$ receptor antagonists that act as channel blockers and negative modulators that do not produce convulsions in vivo. Explanation of this apparent paradox includes selective actions on $GABA_A$ receptor subtypes, reduction of glutamate release from presynaptic terminals via presynaptic receptors and effects on GABA metabolism, together with actions on non-GABAergic systems.

Owing to their unique characteristics, bilobalide and other natural terpenoids from *Gingko biloba* are being investigated as cognitive enhancers via their effects on the GABAergic system [61]. Bilobalide has been shown to improve cognition in cognitive- and memory-impaired animals in a variety of animal models [62–65]. As a result to its nonconvulsant effects, bilobalide is a superior candidate for therapeutic use in memory impairment related to dementia and other neurological disorders compared with other $GABA_A$ receptor antagonists like picrotoxin which are pro-convulsive. Natural terpenoids from *Gingko biloba*, such as bilobalide, are being investigated in the treatment of neurological disorders via their effects on the GABAergic system [61].

The plant-derived triterpenoids, asiatic, oleanolic, and ursolic acids (**Figure 2**), are negative modulators of $GABA_A$ receptor activation acting in vivo as anxiolytics, anticonvulsants, and antidepressants in animal models [66, 67].

7. S44819, an α5-selective competitive antagonist

The α-β subunit interface has been highlighted as a novel target for subtype-selective drugs [68]. An example of a novel drug that targets this binding site and that is attracting considerable current attention as a new therapeutic agent is S44819 (Egis-13,529, 8-Methyl-5-[4-(trifluoromethyl)-1-benzothiophen-2-yl]-1,9-dihydro-2H-[1,3]oxazolo[4,5-h][2,3]benzodiazepin-2-one, **Figure 2**), a novel oxazolo-2,3-benzodiazepine derivative, which selectively inhibits $GABA_A$ receptors that contain the α5-subunit [69, 70].

S44819 appears to act as a competitive antagonist at the orthosteric site at the α-β subunit interface of $GABA_A$ receptors containing only α5 subunits. Thus, S44819 is a competitive antagonist, unlike other α5-subunit selective drugs that act as negative allosteric modulators by binding to the benzodiazepine recognition site between at the α5-γ2 subunits [71, 72]. Agents that are selective for α5 subunit-containing $GABA_A$ receptors enhance cognitive performance in a variety of animal models without sedative or pro-convulsive effects [73]. SR44819 has been shown in healthy young humans to be orally active, reaching the cerebral cortex on oral administration where it increases cortical excitability [74], acting on extrasynaptic receptors to reduce tonic inhibition. Consequently, clinical trials are now underway.

8. Other GABA receptor antagonists

It has not been possible to cover all known GABA receptor antagonists in this perspective. Other important classes of antagonists include sulfated neurosteroids [75] and agents derived from 4-PIOL (5-(4-piperidyl)isoxazol-3-ol) [5]. Of particular interest is DPP-4-PIOL (4-(3,3-diphenylpropyl)-5-(4-piperidyl)-3-isoxazolol hydrobromide) that selectively antagonizes tonic over phasic GABAergic currents in the hippocampus, suggesting a degree of substrate specificity [76].

http://dx.doi.org/10.5772/intechopen.72678

Salicylidene salicylhydrazide has been reported as a potent antagonist of $GABA_A$ receptors containing the β1 subunit using a high-throughput screen [77]. It was suggested that salicylidene salicylhydrazide is interacting at a previously unidentified site on the β1 subunit, but this does not appear to have been followed up after the initial publication in 2004.

The most potent $GABA_A$ receptor antagonist is the convulsant steroid derivative RU5135, being some 500 times more potent than bicuculline [78]. It acts as a competitive antagonist, sharing a common site of action with bicuculline. However it lacks specificity, as it is also a glycine receptor antagonist sharing a common site of action with strychnine [79].

9. Conclusion

There is still widespread interest in GABA receptor antagonists after many years of investigation. Reflecting on the use of GABA receptor antagonists in the last 10 years, citation counts via the Web of Science for publications citing GABA together with a GABA antagonist in the title or abstract are as follows: bicuculline 1203, picrotoxin or picrotoxinin 564, gabazine or SR 95531 290, TPMPA 48, and bilobalide 14. Thus far, there are only four publications directly related to the effects of S44819 on cognition.

Nonconvulsant antagonists of ionotropic GABA receptors have considerable therapeutic potential in the treatment of cognitive problems, myopia, and other CNS disorders. Such antagonists may be useful in the treatment of Down syndrome [62]. The myriad of possible subtypes of ionotropic GABA receptors in the CNS as a result of different combinations of protein subunits make the search for more subtype-specific agents highly desirable. The high-throughput analysis of ionotropic GABA receptor subtypes should result in the discovery of novel subtype-specific agonists, antagonists, and modulators that have therapeutic potential [80]. Clearly, we are going to hear a lot more about S44819 and other yet to be discovered ionotropic GABA receptor antagonists that act selectively on ionotropic GABA receptor subtypes.

Acknowledgements

The authors are grateful to Dr. Ken Mewett for helpful comments.

Author details

Tina Hinton and Graham A. R. Johnston*

*Address all correspondence to: graham.johnston@sydney.edu.au

School of Medical Sciences (Pharmacology), The University of Sydney, Sydney, NSW, Australia

References

[1] Editorial. Advantages of an antagonist. Nature. 1970;**226**:1199-200

[2] Curtis DR, Duggan AW, Felix D, Johnston GAR. GABA, bicuculline and central inhibition. Nature. 1970;**226**:1222-1224

[3] Johnston GAR. Advantages of an antagonist: Bicuculline and other GABA antagonists. British Journal of Pharmacology. 2013;**169**:328-336

[4] Bowery NG, Smart TG. GABA and glycine as neurotransmitters: A brief history. British Journal of Pharmacology. 2006;**147**(Suppl 1):S109-S119

[5] Krall J, Balle T, Krogsgaard-Larsen N, Sorensen TE, Krogsgaard-Larsen P, Kristiansen U, et al. $GABA_A$ receptor partial agonists and antagonists: Structure, binding mode, and pharmacology. Advances in Pharmacology. 2015;**72**:201-227

[6] Hill DR, Bowery NG. ^{3}H-baclofen and ^{3}H-GABA bind to bicuculline insensitive GABA sites in rat brain. Nature. 1981;**290**:149-152

[7] Chebib M, Johnston GAR. GABA-activated ligand gated ion channels: Medicinal chemistry and molecular biology. Journal of Medicinal Chemistry. 2000;**43**:1427-1447

[8] Pritchett DB, Sontheimer H, Shivers BD, Ymer S, Kettenmann H, Schofield PR, et al. Importance of a novel GABAa receptor subunit for benzodiazepine pharmacology. Nature. 1989;**338**:582-585

[9] Thompson SA, Whiting PJ, Wafford KA. Barbiturate interactions at the human $GABA_A$ receptor: Dependence on receptor subunit combination. British Journal of Pharmacology. 1996;**117**:521-527

[10] Belelli D, Casula A, Ling A, Lambert JJ. The influence of subunit composition on the interaction of neurosteroids with $GABA_A$ receptors. Neuropharmacology. 2002;**43**:651-661

[11] Belelli D, Lambert JJ. Neurosteroids: Endogenous regulators of the GABA(a) receptor. Nature Reviews Neuroscience. 2005;**6**:565-575

[12] Mihalek RM, Banerjee PK, Korpi ER, Quinlan JJ, Firestone LL, Mi ZP, et al. Attenuated sensitivity to neuroactive steroids in γ-aminobutyrate type a receptor delta subunit knockout mice. Proceedings of the National Academy of Sciences of the United States of America. 1999;**96**:12905-12910

[13] Gong P, Hong H, Perkins EJ. Ionotropic GABA receptor antagonism-induced adverse outcome pathways for potential neurotoxicity biomarkers. Biomarkers in Medicine. 2015;**9**:1225-1239

[14] Eccles JC, Willis WD, Schmidt R. Pharmacological studies on presynaptic inhibition. Journal of Physiology (London). 1963;**168**:500-530

[15] Davidoff RA, Aprison MH. Picrotoxin antagonism of the inhibition of interneurones by glycine. Life Sciences. 1968;**8**:107-112

[16] Curtis DR, Duggan AW, Johnston GAR. Glycine, strychnine, picrotoxin and spinal inhibition. Brain Research. 1969;**14**:759-762

[17] Krishek BJ, Moss SJ, Smart TGA. Functional comparison of the antagonists bicuculline and picrotoxin at recombinant $GABA_A$ receptors. Neuropharmacology. 1996;**35**:1289-1298

[18] Thompson AJ, Lester HA, Lummis SCR. The structural basis of function in Cys-loop receptors. Quarterly Reviews of Biophysics. 2010;**43**:449-499

[19] Curtis DR, Davies J, Game CJ, Johnston GAR, McCulloch RM. Central actions of shikimin and tutin. Brain Research. 1973;**63**:419-423

[20] Fastier FN, Laws GF. Drugs from New Zealand plants. Search. 1975;**6**:117-120

[21] Curtis DR, Hosli L, Johnston GAR. Inhibition of spinal neurones by glycine. Nature. 1967;**215**:1502-1503

[22] Curtis DR, Duggan AW, Felix D, Johnston GAR. Bicuculline and central GABA receptors. Nature. 1970;**228**:676-677

[23] Ebert B, Thompson SA, Saounatsou K, McKernan R, Krogsgaard-Larsen P, Wafford KA. Differences in agonist/antagonist binding affinity and receptor transduction using recombinant human γ-aminobutyric acid type a receptors. Molecular Pharmacology. 1997; **52**:1150-1156

[24] Andrews PR, Johnston GAR. GABA agonists and antagonists. Biochemical Pharmacology. 1979;**28**:2697-2702

[25] Macdonald RL, Rogers CJ, Twyman RE. Kinetic properties of the $GABA_A$ receptor main conductance state of mouse spinal cord neurones in culture. Journal of Physiology. 1989; **419**:479-499

[26] Olsen RW, Ban M, Miller T, Johnston GAR. Chemical instability of the GABA antagonist bicuculline under physiological conditions. Brain Research. 1975;**98**:383-387

[27] Pong SF, Graham LT. N-methyl bicuculline, a convulsant more potent than bicuculline. Brain Research. 1972;**42**:486-490

[28] Johnston GAR, Beart PM, Curtis DR, Game CJ, McCulloch RM, Maclachlan RM. Bicuculline methochloride as a GABA antagonist. Nature: New Biology. 1972;**240**:219-220

[29] Seutin V, Johnson SW. Recent advances in the pharmacology of quaternary salts of bicuculline. Trends in Pharmacological Sciences. 1999;**20**:268-270

[30] Demuro A, Palma E, Eusebi F, Miledi R. Inhibition of nicotinic acetylcholine receptors by bicuculline. Neuropharmacology. 2001;**41**:854-861

[31] Breuker E, Johnston GAR. Inhibition of acetylcholinesterase by bicuculline and related alkaloids. Journal of Neurochemistry. 1975;**25**:903-904

[32] Ramerstorfer J, Foppa V, Thiery H, Hermange P, Janody S, Berger ML, et al. GABA(a) receptor subtype-selectivity of novel bicuculline derivatives. Current Medicinal Chemistry. 2015;**22**:771-780

[33] Majd AM, Tabar FE, Afghani A, Ashrafpour S, Dehghan S, Gol M, et al. Inhibition of GABA a receptor improved special memory impairment in the local model of demyelination in rat hippocampus. Behavioural Brain Research. 2018;**336**:111-121

[34] Heaulme M, Chambion JP, Leyris R, MJ C, Wermuth CG, Bizuere K. Biochemical characterization of the interaction of three pridazinyl-GABA derivates with the $GABA_A$ receptor site. Brain Research. 1986;**384**:224-231

[35] Uchida I, Cestari IN, Yang J. The differential antagonism by bicuculline and SR95531 of pentobarbitone-induced currents un cultured hippocampal neurons. European Journal of Pharmacology. 1996;**307**:89-96

[36] Ueno S, Bracamontes J, Zorumski C, Weiss DS, Steinbach JH. Bicuculline and gabazine are allosteric inhibitors of channel opening of the $GABA_A$ receptor. Journal of Neuroscience. 1997;**17**:625-634

[37] Yamamoto I, Carland JE, Locock K, Gavande N, Absalom N, Hanrahan JR, et al. Structurally diverse GABA antagonists interact differently with open and closed conformational states of the ρ1 receptor. ACS Chemical Neuroscience. 2012;**3**:293-301

[38] Lee HJ, Absalom NL, Hanrahan JR, van Nieuwenhuijzen P, Ahring PK, Chebib M. A pharmacological characterization of GABA, THIP and DS2 at binary alpha4beta3 and beta3delta receptors: GABA activates beta3delta receptors via the beta3(+)delta(-) interface. Brain Research. 2016:**1644**;222-230

[39] Iqbal F, Ellwood R, Mortensen M, Smart TG, Baker JR. Synthesis and evaluation of highly potent $GABA_A$ receptor antagonists based on gabazine (SR-95531). Bioorganic & Medicinal Chemistry Letters. 2011;**21**:4252-4254

[40] Mortensen M, Iqbal F, Pandurangan AP, Hannan S, Huckvale R, Topf M, et al. Photo-antagonism of the $GABA_A$ receptor. Nature Communications. 2014;**5**:4454

[41] Naffaa MM, Hung S, Chebib M, Johnston GAR, Hanrahan JR. GABA-r receptors: Distinctive functions and molecular pharmacology. British Journal of Pharmacology. 2017; **174**:1881-1894

[42] Johnston GAR, Chebib M, Hanrahan JR, Mewett KN. $GABA_C$ receptors as drug targets. Current Drug Targets. CNS and Neurological Disorders. 2003;**2**:260-268

[43] Murata Y, Woodward RM, Miledi R, Overman LE. The first selective antagonist for a $GABA_C$ receptor. Bioorganic & Medicinal Chemistry Letters. 1996;**6**:2073-2076

[44] Ragozzino D, Woodward RM, Murata Y, Eusebi F, Overman LE, Miledi R. Design and in vitro pharmacology of a selective γ-aminobutyric $acid_C$ receptor antagonist. Molecular Pharmacology. 1996;**50**:1024-1030

[45] Krogsgaard-Larsen P, Johnston GAR, Lodge D, Curtis DR. A new class of GABA agonist. Nature. 1977;**268**:53-55

[46] Krehan D, Frølund B, Krogsgaard-Larsen P, Kehler J, Johnston GAR, Chebib M. Phosphinic, phosphonic and seleninic acid bioisosteres of isonipecotic acid as novel and selective $GABA_C$ receptor antagonists. Neurochemistry International. 2003;**42**:561-565

[47] Locock KE, Yamamoto I, Tran P, Hanrahan JR, Chebib M, Johnston GAR, et al. γ-aminobutyric acid(C) (GABAC) selective antagonists derived from the bioisosteric modification of 4-aminocyclopent-1-enecarboxylic acid: Amides and hydroxamates. Journal of Medicinal Chemistry. 2013;**56**:5626-5630

[48] Pasternack M, Boller M, Pau B, Schmidt M. $GABA_A$ and $GABA_C$ receptors have contrasting effects on excitability in superior colliculus. Journal of Neurophysiology. 1999;**82**:2020-2023

[49] Gibbs ME, Johnston GAR. Opposing roles for $GABA_A$ and $GABA_C$ receptors in short-term memory formation in young chicks. Neuroscience. 2005;**131**:567-576

[50] Chebib M, Hinton T, Schmid KL, Brinkworth D, Qian H, Matos S, et al. Novel, potent, and selective $GABA_C$ antagonists inhibit myopia development and facilitate learning and memory. Journal of Pharmacology and Experimental Therapeutics. 2009;**328**:448-457

[51] Cheng ZY, Wang XP, Schmid KL, Han XG. Inhibition of form-deprivation myopia by a $GABA_A$Or receptor antagonist, (1,2,5,6-tetrahydropyridin-4-yl) methylphosphinic acid (TPMPA), in guinea pigs. Graefes Archive for Clinical and Experimental Ophthalmology. 2014;**252**:1939-1946

[52] Froestl W, Markstein R, Schmid KL, Trendelenburg A-U. GABAc antagonists for the treatment of myopia. PCT International Application. 2004;20030627

[53] Mohammadi E, Shamsizadeh A, Salari E, Fatemi I, Allahtavakoli M, Roohbakhsh A. Effect of TPMPA (GABA(C) receptor antagonist) on neuronal response properties in rat barrel cortex. Somatosensory & Motor Research. 2017;**34**:108-115

[54] Cunha C, Monfils MH, LeDoux JE. GABA(C) receptors in the lateral amygdala: A possible novel target for the treatment of fear and anxiety disorders? Frontiers in Behavioral Neuroscience. 2010;**4**:6. DOI: 10.3389/neuro.08.006.2010

[55] Froestl W. An historical perspective on GABAergic drugs. Future Medicinal Chemistry. 2011;**3**:163-175

[56] Gavande N, Kim HL, Doddareddy MR, Johnston GAR, Chebib M, Hanrahan JR. Design, synthesis, and pharmacological evaluation of fluorescent and biotinylated antagonists of rho(1) GABA(C) receptors. ACS Medicinal Chemistry Letters. 2013;**4**:402-407

[57] Huang SH, Lewis TM, Lummis SCR, Thompson AJ, Chebib M, Johnston GAR, et al. Mixed antagonistic effects of the ginkgolides at recombinant human rho(1) GABA(C) receptors. Neuropharmacology. 2012;**63**:1127-1139

[58] Thompson AJ, Jarvis GE, Duke RK, Johnston GAR, Lummis SC. Ginkgolide B and bilobalide block the pore of the $5\text{-}HT_3$ receptor at a location that overlaps the picrotoxin binding site. Neuropharmacology. 2011;**60**:488-495

[59] Ivic L, Sands TT, Fishkin N, Nakanishi K, Kriegstein AR, Stromgaard K. Terpene trilactones from *Ginkgo biloba* are antagonists of cortical glycine and $GABA_A$ receptors. Journal of Biological Chemistry. 2003;**278**:49279-49285

[60] Ng CC, Duke RK, Hinton T, Johnston GAR. Effects of bilobalide, ginkgolide B and picrotoxinin on GABA(a) receptor modulation by structurally diverse positive modulators. European Journal of Pharmacology. 2017;**806**:83-90

[61] Manayi A, Nabavi SM, Daglia M, Jafari S. Natural terpenoids as a promising source for modulation of GABAergic system and treatment of neurological diseases. Pharmacological Reports. 2016;**68**:671-679

[62] Fernandez F, Morishita W, Zuniga E, Nguyen J, Blank M, Malenka RC, et al. Pharmacotherapy for cognitive impairment in a mouse model of down syndrome. Nature Neuroscience. 2007;**10**:411-413

[63] Li WZ, WY W, Huang H, YY W, Yin YY. Protective effect of bilobalide on learning and memory impairment in rats with vascular dementia. Molecular Medicine Reports. 2013; **8**:935-941

[64] Ma LG, Wang SY, Tai FD, Yuan G, RY W, Liu X, et al. Effects of bilobalide on anxiety, spatial learning, memory and levels of hippocampal glucocorticoid receptors in male Kunming mice. Phytomedicine. 2012;**20**:89-96

[65] Yin YY, Ren YG, Wu WY, Wang YC, Cao MC, Zhu ZY, et al. Protective effects of bilobalide on a beta(25-35) induced learning and memory impairments in male rats. Pharmacology Biochemistry and Behavior. 2013;**106**:77-84

[66] Abdelhalim A, Karim N, Chebib M, Aburjai T, Khan I, Johnston GAR, et al. Antidepressant, anxiolytic and antinociceptive activities of constituents from *Rosmarinus officinalis*. Journal of Pharmacy & Pharmaceutical Sciences. 2015;**18**:448-459

[67] Hamid K, Ng I, Tallapragada VJ, Varadi L, Hibbs DE, Hanrahan J, et al. An investigation of the differential effects of ursane triterpenoids from *Centella asiatica*, and their semisynthetic analogues, on GABA(a) receptors. Chemical Biology & Drug Design. 2016;**88**:386-397

[68] Ramerstorfer J, Furtmuller R, Sarto-Jackson I, Varagic Z, Sieghart W, Ernst M. The $GABA_A$ receptor alpha+beta- interface: A novel target for subtype selective drugs. Journal of Neuroscience. 2011;**31**:870-877

[69] Ling I, Mihalik B, Etherington LA, Kapus G, Palvolgyi A, Gigler G, et al. A novel GABA(a) alpha 5 receptor inhibitor with therapeutic potential. European Journal of Pharmacology. 2015;**764**:497-507

[70] Etherington LA, Mihalik B, Palvolgyi A, Ling I, Pallagi K, Kertesz S, et al. Selective inhibition of extra-synaptic alpha 5-GABA(a) receptors by S44819, a new therapeutic agent. Neuropharmacology. 2017;**125**:353-364

[71] Atack JR. $GABA_A$ receptor subtype-selective modulators. II. alpha5-selective inverse agonists for cognition enhancement. Current Topics in Medicinal Chemistry. 2011;**11**:1203-1214

[72] Braudeau J, Delatour B, Duchon A, Pereira PL, Dauphinot L, de Chaumont F, et al. Specific targeting of the GABA-A receptor alpha5 subtype by a selective inverse agonist

restores cognitive deficits in down syndrome mice. Journal of Psychopharmacology. 2011;**25**:1030-1042

[73] Gacsalyi I, Moricz K, Gigler G, Wellmann J, Nagy K, Ling I, et al. Behavioural pharmacology of the alpha 5-GABA(a) receptor antagonist S44819: Enhancement and remediation of cognitive performance in preclinical models. Neuropharmacology. 2017;**125**:30-38

[74] Darmani G, Zipser CM, Bohmer GM, Deschet K, Muller-Dahlhaus F, Belardinelli P, et al. Effects of the selective alpha5-GABAAR antagonist S44819 on excitability in the human brain: A TMS-EMG and TMS-EEG phase I study. Journal of Neuroscience. 2016; **36**:12312-12320

[75] Chisari M, Wu K, Zorumski CF, Mennerick S. Hydrophobic anions potently and uncompetitively antagonize GABA(a) receptor function in the absence of a conventional binding site. British Journal of Pharmacology. 2011;**164**:667-680

[76] Boddum K, Frolund B, Kristiansen U. The $GABA_A$ antagonist DPP-4-PIOL selectively antagonises tonic over phasic GABAergic currents in dentate gyrus granule cells. Neurochemical Research. 2014;**39**:2078-2084

[77] Thompson SA, Wheat L, Brown NA, Wingrove PB, Pillai GV, Whiting PJ, et al. Salicylidene salicylhydrazide, a selective inhibitor of b1-containing $GABA_A$ receptors. British Journal of Pharmacology. 2004;**142**:97-106

[78] Hunt P, Clementsjewery S. A steroid derivative, R-5135, antagonizes the GABA-benzodiazepine receptor interaction. Neuropharmacology. 1981;**20**:357-361

[79] Simmonds MA, Turner JP. Antagonism of inhibitory amino acids by the steroid derivative RU5135. British Journal of Pharmacology. 1985;**84**:631-635

[80] Nik AM, Pressly B, Singh V, Antrobus S, Hulsizer S, Rogawski MA, et al. Rapid throughput analysis of $GABA_A$ receptor subtype modulators and blockers using DiSBAC1(3) membrane potential red dye. Molecular Pharmacology. 2017;**92**:88-99

Chapter 7

Clinical Application of MR Spectroscopy in Identifying Biochemical Composition of the Intracranial Pathologies

B C Hamsini, Bhavana Nagabhushana Reddy,
Sankar Neelakantan and
Sunitha Palasamudram Kumaran

Additional information is available at the end of the chapter

http://dx.doi.org/10.5772/intechopen.71728

Abstract

Magnetic resonance spectroscopy (MRS) provides useful information regarding metabolic composition in the tissues, and advanced spectroscopic methods are used to quantify markers of tumor membrane turnover and proliferation (e.g., choline (Cho)), energy homoeostasis (e.g., creatine (Cr)), intact glioneuronal structures (e.g., N-acetylaspartate (NAA)), and necrosis (e.g., lactate (Lac) or lipids). Results are usually expressed as metabolite ratios rather than absolute metabolite concentrations. Because glial tumors have some specific metabolic characteristics that differ according to the grade of tumor, there is a potential for MR spectroscopy to increase the sensitivity of routinely used diagnostic imaging. MRS also has many diagnostic applications in neurosciences to support the diagnosis in conditions like demyelination, infections, and dementia and in postradiotherapy cases. Biochemical changes in the metabolism of tumor cells related to malignant transformation are reflected in changes of particular metabolite concentration in the tumor tissue. Our prospective study aimed to analyze the usefulness of proton MR spectroscopy in grading of glioma and to correlate various metabolite ratios like choline/creatine, choline/N-acetylaspartate, N-acetylaspartate/creatine, and lactate/creatine with the histopathological grades of glioma.

Keywords: MRS, MRI, grade, glioma, NAA, choline, creatine, ratio

1. Introduction

Magnetic resonance spectroscopy (MRS) is an analytical method used for the identification and quantification of metabolites. It differs from conventional magnetic resonance imaging (MRI) since it provides physiological and chemical information instead of only anatomy [1].

Many of nuclei have been used to obtain MR spectra; few of them include proton (^{1}H), phosphorus (^{31}P), fluorine (^{19}F), carbon (^{13}C), and sodium (^{23}Na).

Proton (^{1}H) MR spectroscopy is most commonly used since hydrogen nucleus is abundant in human tissues [1].

Magnetic field strength clinically used for conventional MRI ranges from 0.2 to 3 T.

For MRS, higher-field strength (1.5 T or more) is required since the main aim of MRS is to detect weaker signals from metabolites. Higher-field strength units have the advantage of higher signal-to-noise ratio (SNR), better resolution, and shorter acquisition times.

2. Metabolites in MRS

2.1. N-Acetylaspartate (NAA)

N-Acetylaspartate (NAA) peak is the most prominent peak in normal adult brain proton MRS which resonates at 2.0 ppm [2] (**Figure 1**).

NAA is a derivative of aspartic acid. It is synthesized and stored primarily in the neurons and hence it is called a neuronal marker or a marker of neuronal density and viability [2].

As a neuronal marker, NAA concentration declines with the destruction of neurons in high-volume lesions, dementia, hypoxia, or multiple sclerosis.

Due to the relationship between the decline in NAA concentration and increasing glioma grade, it is possible to use NAA as a substantial marker [13]. A high level of NAA is associated with a good prognosis [3].

NAA is also helpful for the differentiation of primary brain tumors from metastasis and non-neuronal tumors where the metabolite is lacking in the spectra [4].

2.2. Creatine (Cr)

Creatine (Cr) is synthesized from amino acids primarily in the kidneys and liver and transported to the peripheral organs by blood and is called as energy metabolism marker [3].

Total Cr indicates the quantity of phosphocreatine (PCr) and Cr contained in neurons and glial cells and visualized as a prominent peak in MR spectra at 3.0 ppm; an additional peak for creatine may be visible at 3.94 ppm [3].

A decrease in the Cr level in high-grade gliomas (HGGs) is due to increased metabolic demands of the tumorous tissue in the brain. Cr is a relatively constant element of cellular energetic metabolism of the brain and it is frequently used as a reference metabolite for in vivo MRS, for example, for mainly calculating the metabolite ratios such as choline (Cho)/Cr, NAA/Cr, lipid (Lip)-lactate (Lac)/Cr, or myoinositol/Cr [3].

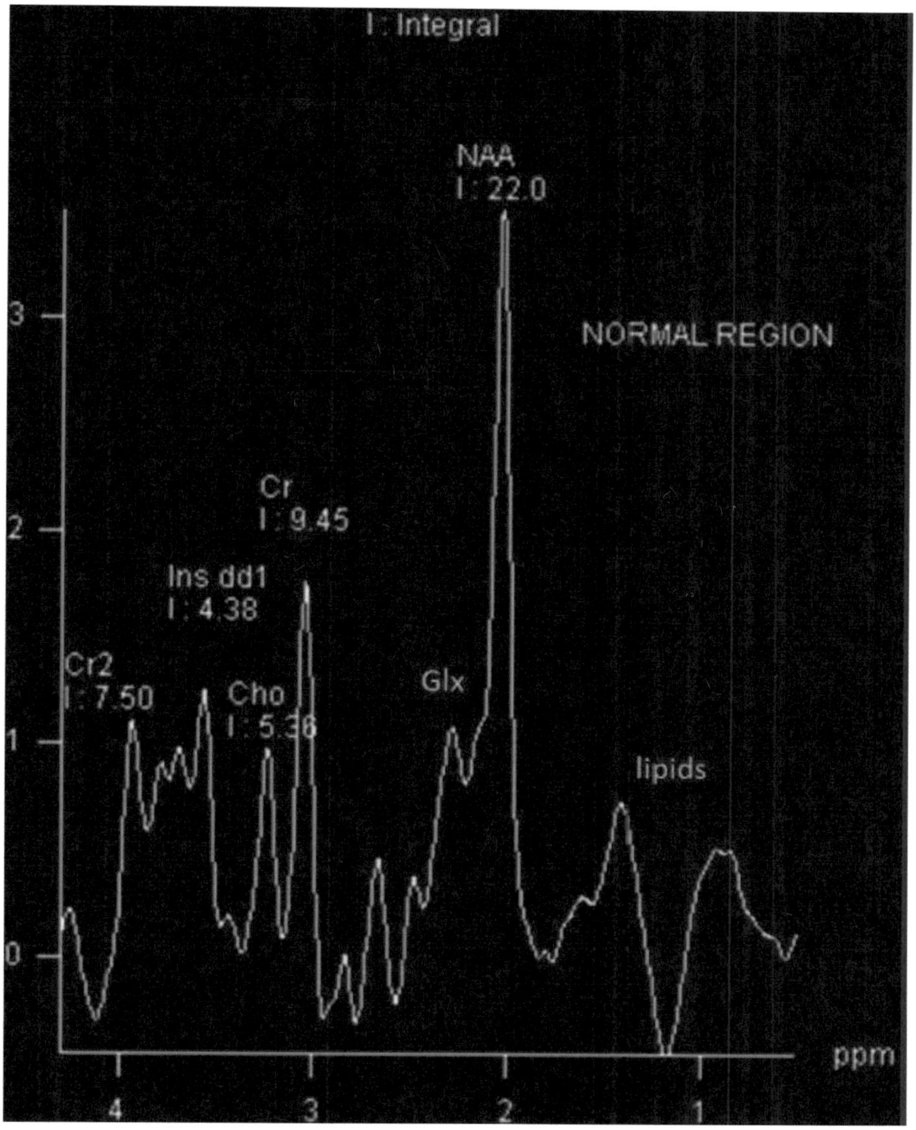

Figure 1. Normal spectra obtained with short TE sequence (TE = 30 ms). Ins dd1, myoinositol; Cho, choline; Cr, creatine; Glx, glutamate glutamine; NAA, N-acetylaspartate [9].

2.3. Choline (Cho)

Choline (Cho) is a metabolic marker of cellular proliferation and cell membrane integrity, that is, phospholipids synthesis and degradation. Choline peak is seen at 3.2 ppm and is the most important metabolic peak for the diagnosis of a glioma [3].

Increased choline reflects increased cell membrane synthesis and degradation. Thus, all processes resulting in increased membrane turnover like primary brain neoplasm and myelin breakdown like demyelinating lesions lead to increased choline concentration [5].

2.4. Myoinositol (Myo)

Myoinositol (Myo) is a simple sugar assigned at 3.56 ppm.

It is considered as a glial marker because it is primarily synthesized in glial cells, almost only in astrocytes. It is also the most important osmolyte in astrocytes [3].

The elevation in Myo detected can be found in cerebral diseases associated with marked gliosis. Myo concentration is higher in low-grade glioma (LGG) when compared to high-grade glioma. Thus, a higher Myo/Cr ratio is seen in low-grade glioma [6].

2.5. Lactate (lac) and lipids (lip)

Lactate (Lac) and lipids (Lip) are known as anaerobic metabolism markers. They are represented as a doublet peak in the MR spectra at 1.31 ppm. It is important to note that lactate is not detected in healthy adult brain tissue. There is direct correlation between Lac level and glioma grade [3].

Malignant transformation of the glial tumors is usually accompanied by an increase in cell density with their relative ischemia resulting in a higher level of Lac. When ischemia of tumorous tissue progresses further, the peaks of Lip increase, indicating the presence of necrosis and the destruction of myelin sheaths [7].

Thus, the level of Lip detected by MRS appears to reflect the severity of tissue damage.

2.6. Glutamate (Glu)-glutamine (Gln) and gamma-amino butyric acid

Glx is a complex peak from glutamate (Glu), glutamine (Gln), and gamma-amino butyric acid (GABA) assigned at 2.05–2.50 ppm [1].

These metabolite peaks are difficult to separate at 1.5 T. Glu is an important excitatory neurotransmitter and plays a role in the redox cycle [8, 9].

An elevated concentration of Gln is found in a few conditions such as hepatic encephalopathy [9].

2.7. Alanine (Ala)

Alanine (Ala) is an amino acid and is a doublet peak assigned at 1.48 ppm.

This peak is located above the baseline in spectra obtained with short or long TE and inverts below the baseline at intermediate TE = 135–144 ms [1].

The function of Ala is uncertain; however, it plays a role in the citric acid cycle. Alanine peak may be obscured by lactate peak [8].

An increased concentration of Ala may occur in oxidative metabolism defects [9].

In tumors, an elevated level of Ala is considered specific for meningiomas [1].

2.8. Other amino acids

In addition to alanine, other amino acids may be seen in various pathologies. Peaks of various amino acids may be seen at many levels, 0.9—valine and 3.6—leucine. Amino acids are also seen in abscesses and neurocysticercosis [10].

3. MRS in tumor grading

This is mainly used for glioma grading. Differentiation between low-grade and high-grade gliomas is important for estimating the prognosis and for therapeutic planning. Proton MRS may indicate the tumor grade with more accuracy because it assesses a larger amount of tissue than what is usually excised during the biopsy.

Gliomas are heterogeneous and their spectra vary depending on the region sampled by MRS. Hence, the region of interest chosen for analysis has a higher influence on the results. Multivoxel spectroscopy is generally considered preferable because it allows metabolic heterogeneity to be evaluated in different components of the tumor.

3.1. Useful metabolites for suggesting the tumor grade

3.1.1. Choline

Statistically significant higher values of Cho/Cr and Cho/NAA are observed in high-grade than in low-grade gliomas.

Although the cutoff values of metabolite ratios for grading of gliomas are not well established, Cho/Cr is the most frequently used ratio. Some institutions use a threshold value of 2.0 for Cho/Cr to differentiate low-grade from high-grade gliomas; others use a cutoff value of 2.5.

Although increased Cho is related to tumor grade, few of grade IV gliomas have lower levels of Cho than grade II or grade III gliomas [11]. This may be due to the presence of necrosis in high-grade tumors, because necrosis is associated with a prominent lipid peak along with the reduction of rest other metabolites [12].

3.1.2. Lipids and lactates

The presence of lipids and lactates correlates with the necrosis in high-grade gliomas. High-grade and low-grade tumors and their margins could be differentiated based on the lactate/lipid peaks.

Lipids peak is also found in metastasis. When lipids peak is observed in solid tumors, lymphoma should also be considered.

An increase in the lipid peak is inversely correlated to prognosis [12].

3.1.3. Myoinositol

Useful information on tumor grade can be obtained by assessing the myo levels at short TE (30–35 ms).

Myo/Cr ratio is typically higher in low-grade than in high-grade gliomas. This may be due to a low mitotic index leading to lack of activation phosphatidylinositol metabolism resulting in the accumulation of myo in low-grade gliomas.

In gliomas without alteration in Cho/Cr ratio, increased levels of Myo have been reported to be useful in the identification of low-grade tumors [12].

3.1.4. NAA and Cr

A greatest reduction in NAA and Cr levels has been observed in higher-grade tumors. As the grade of the tumor increases, NAA/Cr ratio decreases and Cho/NAA ratio increases.

4. Other applications of MRS in brain

4.1. Response to radiotherapy

Differentiation between recurrent brain tumor and radiation change/injury is an important concern in postradiotherapy patients with brain tumors and particularly when fresh contrast-enhancing lesions are seen in previously operated and/or irradiated regions.

Proton MRS is useful in differentiating radiation-induced tissue injury from tumor recurrence. Significantly reduced Cho and Cr levels suggest radiation necrosis; increased lipid and lactate signals can also be seen in necrotic areas.

Increased Cho levels relative to the normal tissue suggest recurrence of the tumor. Cho/Cr and/or Cho/NAA ratios are significantly higher in recurrent tumor than in radiation injury [12].

4.2. Infections

Pyogenic abscess: Amino acid peak at 0.9 ppm is useful in differentiating pyogenic abscess from tumors. Abscess from anaerobic organism in addition has acetate and succinate peaks at 1.9 and 2.4 ppm, respectively [13] .

Tuberculous abscess: Spectra from tuberculous abscess shows lipid-lactate peak at 1.3 ppm. No amino acid peak is observed in tubercular abscess, which helps to differentiate it from pyogenic abscess [14].

Fungal abscess: A spectrum in fungal abscesses shows amino acids and lactate peak along with multiple peaks between 3.6 and 4.0 ppm. These peaks have been assigned to trehalose sugar present in the fungal wall [15].

4.3. Metabolic brain disorder

Proton MR spectroscopy is a useful tool in diagnosing metabolic brain disorders when used as an adjunct to conventional MRI.

In most of the inherited metabolic disorders, MRS findings are abnormal but are not specific for a single metabolic disease or syndrome.

Few metabolic diseases have specific MRS findings, either abnormal elevation or reduction of a single normal peak or detection of abnormal metabolite peak.

Specific MRS patterns are mainly found in Canavan's disease with prominently increased NAA peak and creatine deficiency with a characteristic reduced creatine peak. In nonketotic hyperglycemia, there is an appearance of glycine peak at 3.55 ppm and there is detection of branched-chain amino acids in maple syrup urine disease [16].

4.4. Dementia

Neurodegenerative dementia is characterized by elevated myoinositol and decreased N-acetylaspartate levels.

An increase in myoinositol occurs before the reduction of NAA levels in Alzheimer's disease. An NAA/myo ratio in the posterior cingulate gyri decreases with an increasing burden of Alzheimer's disease.

In patients with mild cognitive impairment, 1H MRS is sensitive in the detection of the pathophysiologic processes associated with the risk of dementia [17].

4.5. Brain ischemia

The characteristic spectroscopic finding in acute brain ischemia is the early appearance of a lactate peak, a decrease of NAA, and a slight increase of choline. Lactate is observed within few minutes following brain ischemia and its concentration reduces in sub-acute phase. The intensity of these peaks in the infracted area is related to the prognosis [18].

4.6. Epilepsy

The role of 1H–MRS in epilepsy is to help in characterizing and localizing the epileptogenic focus, especially in patients with refractory focal epilepsy without clear MR imaging findings.

Temporal lobe epilepsy (TLE) is the most common cause of focal epilepsy; reduction in NAA concentration and NAA/Cho + Cr ratio is observed in TLE, which reflects the neuronal damage [1].

5. Materials and methods

5.1. Study site

The study was conducted at the Department of Radio Diagnosis, Sri Sathya Sai Institute of Higher Medical Sciences, Whitefield, Bangalore 560066.

5.2. Study population

Initially, all patients suspicious for glioma and fulfilling the inclusion and exclusion criteria were imaged with conventional MRI and proton MR spectroscopy. All these patients underwent histopathological examination. Specimens were obtained via surgical resection/biopsy. Patients who had histopathological confirmation of glioma were included in the study. Histopathological grading was done according to WHO classification of brain tumors 2007 [19]. Grades I and II were graded as low-grade and grades III and IV were graded as high-grade tumors.

5.3. Study design

The study design was a prospective study.

5.4. Sample size

$$\text{Sample size} = \frac{Z^2_{1-a/2}\, SD^2}{d^2} \quad (1)$$

where $Z_{1\text{-}a/2}$ is the standard normal variant; SD is the standard deviation of variable; d is the absolute error of precision.

The standard deviation of Cho/Cr for high-grade glioma is 1.92; Cho/Cr ratio is taken because for other ratios the sample size becomes very low. Absolute error of precision was 0.5.

$$\begin{aligned}\text{Sample size} &= (1.96)^2 \times (1.92)^2/0.5 \\ &= 3.8 \times 3.6/0.25 \\ &= 54.72(\text{rounded to } 55)\end{aligned} \quad (2)$$

The minimum sample size was around 55; we have included 70 patients.

5.5. Duration of the study

The duration of study was over a period of 14 months from 01-10-2014, to 01-02-2016.

5.6. Inclusion criteria

- All cases with neuroparenchymal space occupying lesions suspicious for gliomas on MRI.
- All age groups.

- Both male and female patient population.

5.7. Exclusion criteria

- Postoperative and postradiotherapy patients.
- Unavailability of histopathological examination.
- MR spectroscopy with artifact, baseline noise, and uninterruptable spectra.
- MRI contraindicated patients:
  - Patients with cardiac pace maker
  - Patients with aneurysm clips in the brain
  - Patients with a metallic foreign body in the eye
  - Patients with severe claustrophobia
  - Pregnant patients
  - Mentally ill patients.

5.8. Methodology

- Concurrence was taken from the chairman, academic committee, scientific committee, and ethical committee for the study.
- Written informed consent was obtained prior to subject enrolment into the study.
- All the patients were subjected to conventional MRI and proton MR spectroscopy.

5.9. Magnetic resonance imaging

For all patients, initially MR imaging was performed with Siemens 1.5 T Magnetom Aera.

A localizing sagittal T1-weighted image was obtained followed by non-enhanced axial and coronal T2-weighted (4500/102 [TR/TE]), axial fluid-attenuated inversion-recovery (FLAIR, 8500/86/2500 [TR/TE/TI]), and T1-weighted axial (600/9 [TR/TE]) images, Susceptibility weighted imaging (50/40 [TR/TE]). Contrast material-enhanced axial T1-weighted imaging was performed.

5.10. Magnetic resonance spectroscopy

After the conventional MRI volume of interest from the lesion (VOI) was selected from T1 post-contrast images, VOI was selected from the solid part of lesion with edges of the voxel well within the mass and in most of the cases perilesional edema was included within the VOI. VOI was carefully selected so that it will not include areas of hemorrhage or calcification and unintended areas like ventricles, calvarium, and so on.

In our institution, we used Multivoxel MR spectroscopy technique (chemical shift method) at intermediate TE of −135 ms.

A typical VOI consisted of an 8 × 8 cm region placed within a 16 × 16 cm field of view on a 1.5-cm transverse section. A 16 × 16 phase-encoding matrix was used to obtain 8 × 8 arrays of spectra in the VOI, with an in-plane resolution of 1 × 1 cm and a voxel size of 1 × 1 × 1.5 cm^3. The time taken to acquire spectra was around 8 min.

The metabolite peaks were assigned as follows: Cho, 3.22 ppm; Cr, 3.02 ppm; NAA, 2.02 ppm; lactate was identified at 1.33 ppm by its characteristic doublet and inversion at intermediate TE. Lipid peak was demonstrated at 0.9–1.3 ppm without inversion at intermediate TE. Metabolite ratios were obtained for Cho/Cr, Cho/NAA, NAA/Cr, and lactate/Cr. Maximal Cho/Cr, Cho/NAA and lactate/Cr and minimum NAA/Cr ratios were obtained from spectral maps. Lactate/Cr was used instead of lipid-lactate/Cr used by other studies in literature because lipid peak was not consistently seen in most of the cases at intermediate TE.

5.11. Statistical methods

The data collected were entered into a Microsoft excel spreadsheet and analyzed using IBM SPSS Statistics, Version 22 (Armonk, NY: IBM Corp). Descriptive data were presented in the form of frequency, percentage, mean, median, standard deviation, and quartiles. The metabolite ratios of Cho/Cr, Cho/NAA, NAA/Cr, and lactate/Cr were calculated. The metabolite ratios between the low-grade and high-grade gliomas were compared using Mann–Whitney *U*-test. Comparisons of the categorical variables between the two groups were performed using the chi-squared test. Receiver-operating characteristic (ROC) curve analysis was done to evaluate the performance of the metabolite ratios in differentiating high-grade and low-grade gliomas. The area under the ROC curve was calculated to summarize the performance of each metabolite in differentiating the two grades of glioma. The sensitivity, specificity, positive-predictive value (PPV), negative-predictive value (NPV), and diagnostic accuracy with each metabolite were assessed using the cutoff value obtained with minimum C1 error from the ROC analysis. A *P*-value of <0.05 was considered as statistically significant. In the same way, ROC curve analysis was done to evaluate the performance of metabolite ratios in differentiating grade II and grade III glioma. By similar way, sensitivity, specificity, positive-predictive value, negative-predictive value, and diagnostic accuracy with each metabolite were assessed using the cutoff value obtained with minimum C1 error from the ROC analysis in differentiating grade II and grade III gliomas.

6. Results

Seventy histopathologically proved cases of gliomas were included in the study. Grade I [14] and grade II [19] gliomas were classified as low-grade and grade III [22] and grade IV [15] were classified as high-grade tumors.

All patients underwent conventional MRI sequences and proton MR spectroscopy. Quantitative values were calculated for Cho/Cr, Cho/NAA, NAA/Cr, and lactate/Cr ratios. Grading by conventional MRI was also done to know the additional usefulness of MRS in grading of gliomas.

The sensitivity, specificity, PPV, and NPV of conventional MRI in grading of gliomas were 62.2, 78.8, 76.7, and 65%, respectively, with the total diagnostic accuracy of 70%.

The sensitivity, specificity, PPV, and NPV of proton MR spectroscopy in differentiating the grades of glioma were high in comparison to conventional MRI indicating that proton MRS spectroscopy is a useful tool in differentiating grades of glioma.

Lac/Cr ratio had a total diagnostic accuracy of 95.12%. Cho/NAA and Cho/Cr ratios had a total diagnostic accuracy of 88.57 and 88.43%, respectively.

Metabolite ratio that had the highest diagnostic value was lactate/Cr followed by Cho/NAA and Cho/Cr in differentiating low- and high-grade gliomas.

NAA/Cr ratio had poor diagnostic significance in differentiating the grades of gliomas.

The presence of lipid peak was found to be suggestive of high-grade gliomas and was found in about 46% of high-grade gliomas.

Other metabolite peaks like myoinositol and glutamate could not be evaluated.

MRS had the added advantage in combination with conventional MRI with good diagnostic accuracy in differentiating grade II and grade III gliomas. Lactate/Cr had the highest diagnostic value followed by Cho/NAA and Cho/Cr in differentiating the two grades.

7. Discussion

Tumor grade is the most important key factor in determining treatment plan. Treatment plan for low-grade glioma is surgical resection; adjuvant radio chemotherapy is only recommended for patients with incompletely resected grade II tumors or for patients older than age of 40 years. Whereas high-grade glioma always require chemotherapy and/or radiotherapy following surgery; therefore, preoperative grading of glioma is necessary for good patient care and to reduce the morbidity and mortality [19].

The current "gold standard" for the determination of glioma grade is histopathological examination. It has few limitations; the most significant one is limited number of samples which creates potential errors in determining the glioma grade. When samples are not taken from the most malignant region of tumor during biopsy or when the tumor has not been completely resected, histopathological grading becomes inaccurate. This problem is particularly observed in glioma because of the infiltrative and heterogeneous nature of these tumors; the region of highest malignancy may then be within the peritumoral or perilesional-enhancing region [20, 21].

Because histopathological examination requires biopsy/surgical resection which are invasive, it has morbidity of up to 3.6%, hemorrhage rate of up to 8%, and mortality of up to 1.7%, as assessed over a large number of studies [22].

Alternatively, many noninvasive or minimally invasive imaging technologies have been used to evaluate the malignancy of brain tumors [20, 21].

In our study, grades I and II were graded as low grade and grades III and IV were graded as high grade [19].

We have used the following criteria for grading gliomas by conventional MRI: margins of the lesion, perilesional edema, heterogeneity of lesion, mass effect, crossing the midline, hemorrhage, necrosis, and enhancement pattern. Other studies have also used the similar criteria [21].

Sensitivity, specificity, PPV, and NPV of conventional MRI in grading of gliomas were found to be 62.2, 78.8, 76.7, and 65%, respectively, with the total diagnostic accuracy of 70%.

In other studies conducted by Law et al. [21], Zou et al. [19], and Ellika et al. [23], the sensitivity ranged from 72 to 86% and the specificity ranged from 60 to 67%.

Other studies in literature have shown sensitivity ranging from 55 to 83% [19, 21].

A study conducted by Dean et al. [24] and Atkinson et al. [25] showed that a high-grade glioma may be mistaken for a low-grade when it demonstrates minimal edema, no contrast enhancement, no necrosis, and no mass effect. Conversely, low-grade gliomas sometimes can be mistaken for a high-grade when it demonstrates peritumoral edema, contrast material enhancement, central necrosis, and mass effect.

Low diagnostic accuracy in our study was because of the overlapping imaging features in low- and high-grade gliomas, predominantly between grades II and grade III. Fourteen cases of grade III tumors were classified as low grade because they had imaging features favoring low grade such as minimal perilesional edema, no significant mass effect, no contrast enhancement, no necrosis, and no hemorrhage.

Seven cases of low-grade gliomas were classified as high grade since they had imaging features favoring high grade such as significant perilesional edema, mass effect, presence of necrosis or hemorrhage, and heterogeneous contrast enhancement.

In our study, the most consistent characteristics on MRI to predict the grade were necrosis, mass effect, and crossing the midline.

A study conducted by Dean et al. [24] has shown that mass effect and necrosis are the most important characteristic for predicting tumor grade by conventional MRI.

Because of the limitations of conventional MRI in differentiating high- from low-grade gliomas, advanced multi-parametric magnetic resonance techniques have been used in grading of gliomas and they are diffusion-weighted imaging (DWI), proton MR spectroscopy, and perfusion imaging [19].

Magnetic resonance spectroscopy is one of the advanced adjuvant MR techniques and because of its safe and noninvasive nature it is of great advantage in characterizing gliomas.

Because glial tumors have some specific metabolic characteristics which further differ according to the grade, there is growing interest in MR spectroscopy that could further increase the sensitivity of routinely used diagnostic imaging [3].

In our study, we have used Cho/Cr, Cho/NAA, NAA/Cr, and lactate/Cr ratios for grading since the study was done at intermediate TE, prominent peaks seen were Cho, Cr, NAA, and lactate.

In literature, Cho/Cr, Cho/NAA, and NAA/Cr were the commonly used metabolites [19, 21]. Lipid-lactate ratio was used for grading of gliomas in few studies [26]; we have used lactate/Cr ration since lipid peak was not consistently seen in a majority of cases at intermediate TE.

In our study, the values of mean and median for Cho/Cr, Cho/NAA, and NAA/Cr had statistically significant difference between low- and high-grade gliomas.

Other studies have also shown significant difference of mean for Cho/Cr, Cho/NAA, and NAA/Cr between low- and high-grade gliomas [10].

NAA is a neuronal marker and decreases in all gliomas since the neurons are destroyed and/or substituted by the malignant cells. The elevation of choline is due to the increased cellularity and cell membrane turnover. The decrease in creatine is due to the altered energy metabolism in the cells and can be attributed to the low energy status of the glycolyzing tumors. Therefore, the typical MRS characteristics of a glioma are elevated Cho with reduction in NAA and Cr signals. This results in an absolute increase in Cho/Cr and Cho/NAA and a decrease in NAA/Cr ratios [1].

Lac/Cr ratio in our study had significant difference in mean between low- and high-grade gliomas.

Studies conducted by Yoon et al. [26] and Kim et al. [27] showed significant difference in mean values for lipid-lactate/Cr between low- and high-grade gliomas.

Since lactate is a marker of anaerobic glycolysis, malignant transformation of glial tumors is accompanied by an increase in cell density with relative ischemia resulting in a higher level of lactate. There is a direct correlation between Lac levels and glioma grade with higher peaks seen in higher-grade tumors [3]. Therefore, Lac/Cr ratio increases with an increase in the malignant potential of tumor.

In a clinical setting, where decisions such as the extent of tumor resection, the dose of post-operative chemo radiation, and the interval of follow-up must be made, cutoff values can be used as important supplementary information in noninvasive grading of gliomas [21].

In our study, we have provided cutoff values for Cho/Cr, Cho/NAA, and lactate/Cr ratios to differentiate low- from high-grade gliomas.

A cutoff value of 1.76 for Cho/Cr and 2.22 for Cho/NAA ratio provided good sensitivity, specificity, PPV, and NPV with a total diagnostic accuracy of 78.05 and 82.93%, respectively, in differentiating low- from high-grade gliomas.

Other studies in literature have given a cutoff value ranging from 1.56 to 2.04 for Cho/Cr and 1.6 to 2.49 for Cho/NAA. These values provided good sensitivity, specificity, PPV, and NPV with a total diagnostic accuracy ranging from 81 to 88% [21].

Even though the cutoff value for Cho/Cr and Cho/NAA provided by our study was comparable with other studies in literature [21], the small variation in cutoff value between studies is possibly because of differences in the MRS imaging methods, including magnetic resonance field strength, acquisition parameters, voxel size and location, heterogeneity of tumor, and sample size and distribution.

A cutoff value of 0.68 for Lac/Cr ratio provided an excellent diagnostic accuracy of 95.12% which was the most useful metabolite ratio in differentiating low- from high-grade gliomas in our study.

Limited studies in literature have given cutoff for lipid-lactate/Cr ratio in grading of gliomas. A study performed by Kim et al. gave a cutoff value of 0.59 for lipid-lactate/Cr [28]. A study performed by Yoon et al. gave a cutoff of 1.39 with a sensitivity of 64.6% and a specificity of 91.7% [26].

There was no cutoff value given for NAA/Cr ratio in our study even though the mean values were statistically significant in differentiating high- and low-grade gliomas because of overlapping of NAA/Cr values between the grades; out of 37 people in high-grade gliomas, 29 (78% of high-grade glioma cases) had values higher than the lowest value in low grade.

Zeng et al. [28] and Liu et al. [29] have given cutoff values of 0.72 and 0.97 for NAA/Cr ratio to differentiate low- and high-grade gliomas with a diagnostic accuracy of 73–75%.

In our study, lipid peak was found in 46% of high-grade and 12% of low-grade gliomas. A prominent lipid peak in high-grade gliomas was due to necrotic component.

Other studies have also shown that gliomas are heterogeneous tumors and they include areas of viable tumor, necrosis, and hemorrhage. Elevated lipid peaks are often found in high-grade gliomas due to the necrotic portion [30, 31].

Since our study is carried out at intermediate TE (135 ms), we could not evaluate other peaks like myoinositol and glutamate. Few cases had myoinositol peak but the peak was not consistently seen to comment upon.

Differentiation between grade II and III gliomas is clinically important since the treatment plan and prognosis are different but it is difficult to differentiate them on conventional MRI because of the overlapping imaging characteristics [32].

Literature review showed limited studies to differentiate grade II and grade III gliomas. In our study, we analyzed and tried to establish cutoff values to differentiate grade II and grade III gliomas.

Lactate/Cr had excellent diagnostic value followed by Cho/NAA and Cho/Cr ratios. NAA/Cr had poor diagnostic value in differentiating the grade II and grade III because of the overlapping of values.

Cutoff values for Cho/Cr, Cho/NAA, and lactate/Cr ratios were 1.76, 2.22, and 0.685 with good sensitivity, specificity, PPV, and NPV. Diagnostic accuracy was 78.05, 82.93, and 95.12% for Cho/Cr, Cho/NAA, and lactate/Cr, respectively.

Stadlbauer et al. [23] found that there was significant difference in Cho, Cr, and NAA levels between grade II and grade III gliomas, and all patients with a grade II glioma had a Cho/NAA ratio of less than 0.8, whereas all patients with a grade III glioma had a Cho/NAA ratio of greater than 0.8.

Zonari et al. [33] found the sensitivity, specificity, PPV, and NPV for Cho/Cr ratio to be 75.6 45, 60.7, and 62.1 and NAA/Cr ratio to be 64.4, 65, 67.4, and 61.9 in differentiating grade II from grade III gliomas by a logistic regression analysis.

Advanced multi-parametric magnetic resonance techniques, including DWI, DTI, and MR perfusion and multimodal imaging including PET/SPECT, also compliment MRS to distinguish HGGs from LGGs. Though it is controversial which imaging technique is superior, most authors concluded that combined techniques would improve the diagnostic accuracy [19].

8. Limitations

1. Our study was done at a magnetic field strength of 1.5 T. A higher-field strength of 3 T or more would have yielded a better spatial resolution and high SNR.
2. Small sample size may reduce or bias the power of the results. Further studies with a larger sample size are necessary to extend these results.
3. Our sample volume predominantly consists of astrocytomas, and other glial tumors like oligodendrogliomas and ependymomas were less frequent.
4. Our study was carried at intermediate TE, so we could not evaluate smaller metabolite peaks like myoinositol and glutamate. MRS at short TE would have given spectra with multiple metabolite peaks.
5. Comparison of MRS with other advanced MR techniques like perfusion and DTI would have given additional value in grading of gliomas.

9. Conclusion

MRS is an important diagnostic and research tool in clinical neuroscience. MRS is a very useful tool in combination with conventional MRI for grading of gliomas. Lactate/creatine ratio has highest diagnostic accuracy followed by choline/NAA and choline/creatine ratios. NAA/creatine has least diagnostic significance in grading of gliomas. Lipid peak on MRS is more frequently found in high-grade gliomas. MRS could differentiate grade II and grade III gliomas more effectively in comparison to only conventional MRI. Apart from tumor grading, MRS can support the diagnosis in many brain infections by showing the specific metabolite peaks. It is also helpful in diagnosis of post-radiotherapy patients when differentiation between recurrent brain tumor and radiation change/injury is the concern. It also has a significant role in narrowing the differential diagnosis of metabolic brain disorders. MRS is also important in the diagnosis of stroke and demyelination in brain.

A. Appendix A

A.1. Representative cases

Case 1. A 46-year-old female presented with headache since 1 year.

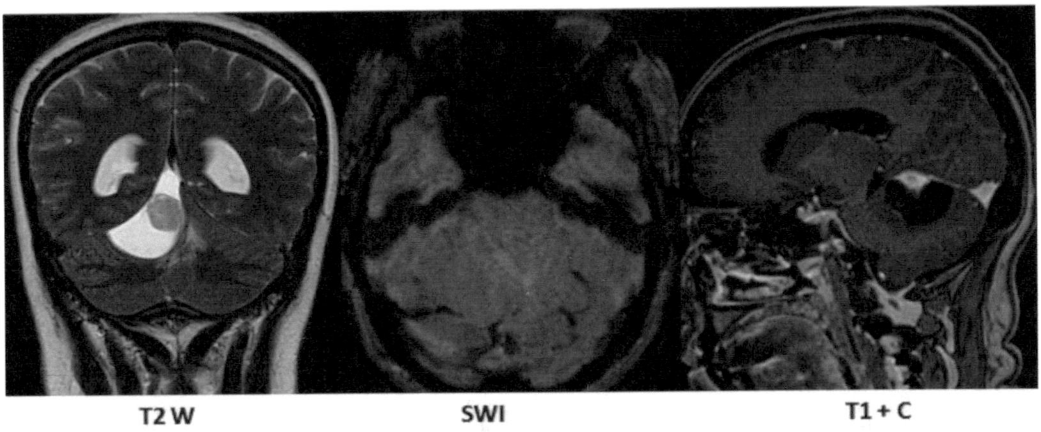

MRI shows well-defined cystic lesion with enhancing peripheral mural nodule in the right cerebellar hemisphere with mild perilesional edema. Local mass effect on the adjacent neuroparenchyma. No areas of hemorrhage on SWI. No areas of necrosis.

Diagnosed as low-grade glioma on conventional MRI.

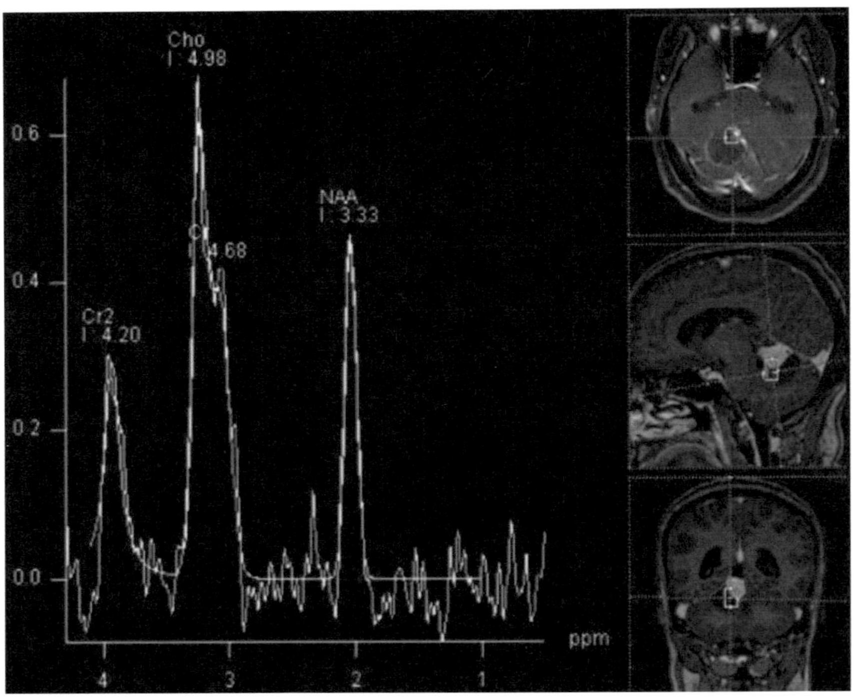

MRS: Elevated choline, reduced NAA, and Cr. Cho/Cr: 1.63; Cho/NAA: 1; NAA/Cr: 1.09; lactate/Cr: 0.18. No lipid peak.

Histopathological diagnosis: Pilocytic astrocytoma (grade I glioma).

http://dx.doi.org/10.5772/intechopen.71728

Case 2: A 70-year-old male presenting with seizures since 2 months.

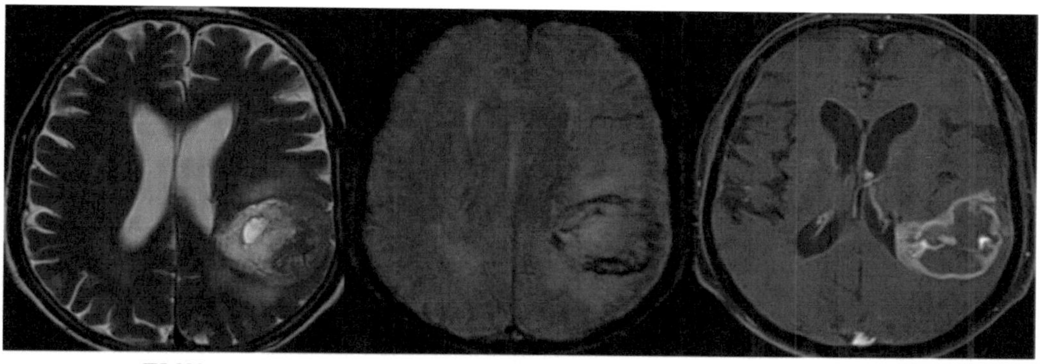

T2 W SWI T1 + C

MRI shows relatively well-defined heterogeneous lesion noted in the left parietal lobe with moderate perilesional edema. There is mass effect on the adjacent neuroparenchyma without midline shift. Areas of necrosis and hemorrhage noted within the lesion. Peripheral nodular enhancement is seen.

Diagnosed as high-grade glioma on conventional MRI.

Relatively well-defined heterogeneous lesion noted in the left parietal lobe with moderate perilesional edema. There is mass effect on the adjacent neuroparenchyma without midline shift. Areas of necrosis and hemorrhage noted within the lesion. Peripheral nodular enhancement is seen.

Diagnosed as high-grade glioma on conventional MRI.

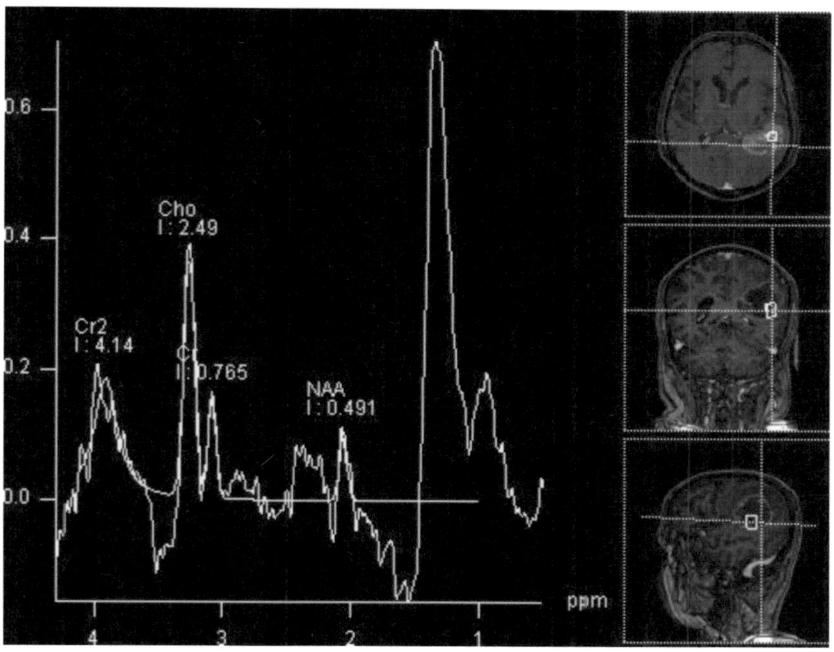

MRS: Elevated choline, reduced NAA, and Cr.

Cho/Cr: 2.47; Cho/NAA: 3.5; NAA/Cr: 0.7; lactate/Cr: 1.

Lipid peak present.

Histopathological diagnosis: GBM (grade IV glioma).

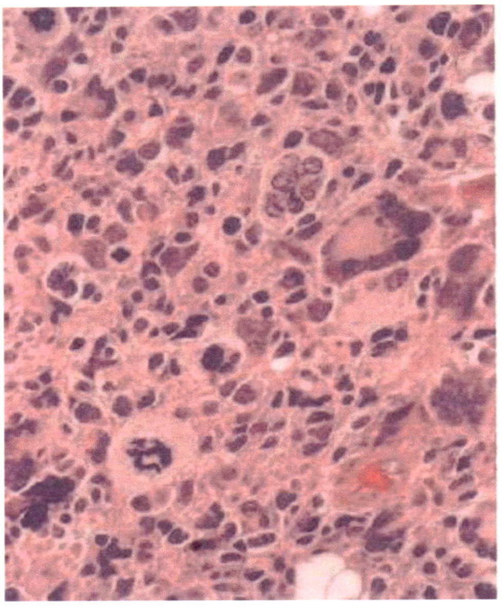

Paraffin section with hematoxylin and eosin stain showing marked nuclear pleomorphism and mitotic figures.

Author details

B C Hamsini[1], Bhavana Nagabhushana Reddy[2], Sankar Neelakantan[2] and Sunitha Palasamudram Kumaran[1,2]*

*Address all correspondence to: drsunitha27@gmail.com

1 Neuroimaging, Toronto Western hospital, Toronto, Ontario, Canada

2 Department of Radiology, Sri Sathya Sai Institute of higher medical sciences, Bangalore, India

References

[1] Bertholdo D, Watcharakorn A, Castillo M. Brain proton magnetic resonance spectroscopy. Neuroimaging Clinics of North America. 2013 Aug;**23**(3):359-380

[2] Smith JK, Castillo M, Kwock L. MR spectroscopy of brain tumors. Magnetic Resonance Imaging Clinics of North America. 2003 Aug;**11**(3):415-429

[3] Bulik M, Jancalek R, Vanicek J, Skoch A, Mechl M. Potential of MR spectroscopy for assessment of glioma grading. Clinical Neurology and Neurosurgery. 2013 Feb;**115**(2):146-153

[4] Young GS. Advanced MRI of adult brain tumors. Neurologic Clinics. 2007 Nov;**25**(4): 947-973

[5] Nelson SJ. Multivoxel magnetic resonance spectroscopy of brain tumors. Molecular Cancer Therapeutics. 2003;**2**(5):497-507

[6] Castillo M, Smith JK, Kwock L. Correlation of myo-inositol levels and grading of cerebral astrocytomas. American Journal of Neuroradiology. 2000 Oct;**21**(9):1645-1649

[7] Yamasaki F, Takaba J, Ohtaki M, Abe N, Kajiwara Y, Saito T, et al. Detection and differentiation of lactate and lipids by single-voxel proton MR spectroscopy. Neurosurgical Review. 2005 Oct;**28**(4):267-277

[8] Soares DP, Law M. Magnetic resonance spectroscopy of the brain: Review of metabolites and clinical applications. Clinical Radiology. 2009 Jan;**64**(1):12-21

[9] Van der Graaf M. In vivo magnetic resonance spectroscopy: Basic methodology and clinical applications. European Biophysics Journal. 2010 Mar;**39**(4):527-540

[10] Chang KH, Song IC, Kim SH, Han MH, Kim HD, Seong SO, et al. In vivo single-voxel proton MR spectroscopy in intracranial cystic masses. American Journal of Neuroradiology. 1998 Mar;**19**(3):401-405

[11] Howe FA, Barton SJ, Cudlip SA, Stubbs M, Saunders DE, Murphy M, et al. Metabolic profiles of human brain tumors using quantitative in vivo 1H magnetic resonance spectroscopy. Magnetic Resonance in Medicine. 2003 Feb;**49**(2):223-232

[12] Brandão LA, Castillo M. Adult brain tumors. Neuroimaging Clinics of North America. 2013 Aug;**23**(3):527-555

[13] Gupta RK, Jobanputra KJ, Yadav A. MR spectroscopy in brain infections. Neuroimaging Clinics of North America. 2013 Aug;**23**(3):475-498

[14] Gupta RK, Vatsal DK, Husain N, Chawla S, Prasad KN, Roy R, et al. Differentiation of tuberculous from pyogenic brain abscesses with in vivo proton MR spectroscopy and magnetization transfer MR imaging. American Journal of Neuroradiology. 2001 Sep; **22**(8):1503-1509

[15] Luthra G, Parihar A, Nath K, Jaiswal S, Prasad KN, Husain N, et al. Comparative evaluation of fungal, tubercular, and pyogenic brain abscesses with conventional and diffusion MR imaging and proton MR spectroscopy. American Journal of Neuroradiology. 2007 Aug;**28**(7):1332-1338

[16] Rossi A, Biancheri R. Magnetic resonance spectroscopy in metabolic disorders. Neuroimaging Clinics of North America. 2013

[17] Kantarci K. Magnetic resonance spectroscopy in common dementias. Neuroimaging Clinics of North America. 2013 Aug;**23**(3):393-406

[18] Ramin SL, Tognola WA, Spotti AR. Proton magnetic resonance spectroscopy: Clinical applications in patients with brain lesions. São Paulo Medical Journal. 2003;**121**(6):254-259

[19] Louis DN, Ohgaki H, Wiestler OD, Cavenee WK, Burger PC, Jouvet A, et al. The 2007 WHO classification of tumours of the central nervous system. Acta Neuropathology (Berl). 2007 Jul 12;**114**(2):97-109

[20] Zou Q-G, Xu H-B, Liu F, Guo W, Kong X-C, Wu Y. In the assessment of supratentorial glioma grade: The combined role of multivoxel proton MR spectroscopy and diffusion tensor imaging. Clinical Radiology. 2011 Oct;**66**(10):953-960

[21] Lu H, Pollack E, Young R, Babb JS, Johnson G, Zagzag D, et al. Predicting grade of cerebral glioma using vascular-space occupancy MR imaging. American Journal of Neuroradiology. 2008 Feb 1;**29**(2):373-378

[22] Law M, Yang S, Wang H, Babb JS, Johnson G, Cha S, et al. Glioma grading: Sensitivity, specificity, and predictive values of perfusion MR imaging and proton MR spectroscopic imaging compared with conventional MR imaging. American Journal of Neuroradiology. 2003;**24**(10):1989-1998

[23] Stadlbauer A, Gruber S, Nimsky C, Fahlbusch R, Hammen T, Buslei R, et al. Preoperative grading of gliomas by using metabolite quanti cation with high-spatial-resolution proton MR spectroscopic imaging 1. Radiology. 2006;**238**(3):958-969

[24] Ellika SK, Jain R, Patel SC, Scarpace L, Schul LR, Rock JP, et al. Role of perfusion CT in glioma grading and comparison with conventional MR imaging features. American Journal of Neuroradiology. 2007 Nov 1;**28**(10):1981-1987

[25] BL DBP, Bird CR, Flom RA, Hodak JA, Coons SW, et al. Gliomas: Classification with MR imaging. Radiology. 1990 Feb;**174**(2):411-415

[26] Atkinson M, Juhász C, Shah J, Guo X, Kupsky W, Fuerst D, et al. Paradoxical imaging findings in cerebral gliomas. Journal of the Neurological Sciences. 2008 Jun;**269**(1-2):180-183

[27] Yoon JH, Kim J, Kang WJ, Sohn C-H, Choi SH, Yun TJ, et al. Grading of cerebral glioma with multiparametric MR imaging and ^{18}F-FDG-PET: Concordance and accuracy. European Radiology. 2014 Feb;**24**(2):380-389

[28] Kim J, Chang K-H, Na DG, Song IC, Kwon BJ, Han MH, et al. 3T 1H-MR spectroscopy in grading of cerebral gliomas: Comparison of short and intermediate echo time sequences. American Journal of Neuroradiology. 2006;**27**(7):1412-1418

[29] Zeng Q, Liu H, Zhang K, Li C, Zhou G. Noninvasive evaluation of cerebral glioma grade by using multivoxel 3D proton MR spectroscopy. Magnetic Resonance Imaging. 2011 Jan;**29**(1):25-31

[30] Liu ZL, Zhou Q, Zeng QS, Li CF, Zhang K. Noninvasive evaluation of cerebral glioma grade by using diffusion-weighted imaging-guided single-voxel proton magnetic resonance spectroscopy. The Journal of International Medical Research. 2012;**40**(1):76-84

[31] Yamasaki F, Takayasu T, Nosaka R, Amatya VJ, Doskaliyev A, Akiyama Y, et al. Magnetic resonance spectroscopy detection of high lipid levels in intraaxial tumors without central necrosis: A characteristic of malignant lymphoma. Journal of Neurosurgery. 2015 Jun;**122**(6):1370-1379

[32] Calvar JA, Meli FJ, Romero C, Yánez MLCP, Martinez AR, Lambre H, et al. Characterization of brain tumors by MRS, DWI and Ki-67 labeling index. Journal of Neuro-Oncology. 2005 May;**72**(3):273-280

[33] Zonari P, Baraldi P, Crisi G. Multimodal MRI in the characterization of glial neoplasms: The combined role of single-voxel MR spectroscopy, diffusion imaging and echo-planar perfusion imaging. Neuroradiology. 2007 Sep 25;**49**(10):795-803